Jack,
Stay Above
Ground *,*

This book is being given to you on behalf of

_____

To clarify any questions regarding the information
contained, please call:

_____

Here's to Aging Healthy, Wealthy & Wisely!

(All rights reserved 2016, Library of Congress)

Published 2016 by Karyn Rizzo All rights reserved.

ISBN

EXPANDED EDITION
Original Print March 2014 "Aging in America What you Need to Know about Navigating our Healthcare System"
ISBN # 978-1-6317340-5-2

This book was printed in the United States of America.

Author Biography

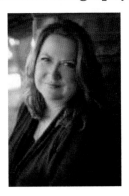

Karyn Rizzo, owner of ELITE Marketing & Consulting has over 20 years of experience working in the Healthcare Industry. A native of Chicago, Illinois, she has lived in Florida and loves the beaches and wonderful weather. She graduated with a degree in Business Management at the University of North Carolina, and subsequently returned to Florida.

Her initial experiences in Physician Administration outlined the challenges physicians face running a practice, as well as the influences of Insurance Companies and our Elected Officials on patient healthcare options and benefits.

Subsequently, working in the Assisted Living and Skilled Nursing Center markets created a unique outlook on the ever changing climate of patient needs and healthcare resources available. Her familiarity with all types of healthcare providers has given her a unique expertise in navigating our healthcare system.

Her passion to help families connect to local resources, receive knowledge and care, has been a key theme of her work over the years. As a patient advocate in every sense, she has worked diligently to protect seniors and their families from those that would take advantage of them for their own personal or financial gain.

She now offers a practical resource guide, "Aging in America Navigating our Healthcare System" (2014 Best Seller), Expanded Edition, written with insider information on the *"BUSINESS"* of Aging in America.

This valuable Resource Guide is available for sale at www.agingguidebook1.com, and on Amazon, Kindle & Nook.

Member, Better Living for Seniors Pinellas / Pasco (BLS)
Member, Bay Area Senior Education Services (BASES)
PR Chair, Advisory Council Member, Retired Senior Volunteer Program (RSVP)

For information discounts, terms and media requests contact:
ELITE Marketing & Consulting
P.O. Box 7221
Seminole, FL 33775
info@agingguidebook1.com

www.agingguidebook1.com

ACKNOWLEDGEMENTS

I would like to dedicate this book to the many confused patients and caregivers that struggle to make the best choices for their loved ones.

And to my devoted husband, *Jason Jimenez,* whose unwavering support is the reason that writing is now a main and constant factor in my life.

I want to dedicate these specific Chapters for the LGBTQ elder to my BFF *Dean Hoffman*, who has been my colleague in healthcare, and a great friend. His openness about his sexuality and the fight for gay rights helped me understand the prejudice and challenges many experience when managing their personal health and wellness as a gay patient.

I'd also like to dedicate this book to the amazing healthcare professionals who treat every patient with the same compassionate care, regardless of diagnosis, sexual orientation, or ethnicity. Your devotion for caring for those in need reflects the best qualities in humanity!

TESTIMONIALS

"Karyn Rizzo provides a great tool for navigating our healthcare system. This practical and easy to read guide gives us the ability to make the right decisions for our own medical care, and the care of our aging family members. Karyn shares with us her remarkable understanding of our constantly changing healthcare system and provides a no-nonsense look at what we can expect and how to plan for our future. "Aging in America" provides websites, phone numbers and advice in selecting the best providers for our plan of care. The information in this guide is invaluable - well done, Karyn!"

Cheryl Wagner, Patient Liaison, Empath Hospice

"The Bay Area Senior Education Services (BASES) is proud to announce the successful launch of a committee member Karyn Rizzo's book on Aging in America. Karyn has done a fantastic job of incorporating the trials and tribulations of America's healthcare system in a more simplistic form. Unlike other books, Aging in America provides solutions to the problems many individuals deal with on a daily basis. Karyn has worked tirelessly with the BASES committee to turn her book into a systematic approach to navigating our healthcare system. We are looking forward to working with Karyn in developing more speaking engagements to continue to promote her vision. You can find her book "AGING in AMERICA; What you need to know about Navigating our Healthcare System" on Amazon, Kindle, Nook and in Barnes & Noble on demand, and at www.agingguidebook1.com. Congratulations Karyn!"

Shane K. Warner, Esq. Elder Law Attorney

"The Aging in America Guidebook is a must read for seniors, families, caregivers, and healthcare professionals. This book is written

in an easy to understand format that will allow the reader to truly understand the resources that are out there for seniors. As a senior healthcare industry professional, I personally endorse this book as a "MUST READ" for anyone dealing with the complexities of Aging in America."

Angela Poirier, Senior Care Professional

"Aging in America is a resource guide that can help the average person understand why the choices they make for healthcare providers is so important. Working with families every day that don't understand the "Business" side of our healthcare, her book is an invaluable tool in helping them understand why they have certain options. I recommend it for anyone with an older loved one."

Dawn Gretter, Sales Counselor Ivy Ridge Inspired Living

"The Resource guide Karyn Rizzo has written for caregiver of elderly people is an excellent tool for families struggling with tough decisions for their loved ones. Often, they are having their own health issues while making important decisions for their loved ones. I'm happy to recommend this resource guide to others that need the help."

Louise Schott, Regional Director, Validus Senior Living

DISCLAIMER

The author of this book does not dispense medical nor prescribe the use of any technique as a form of treatment for physical, emotional, or medical problems without the advice of a physician, either directly or indirectly.

The author does not give legal or financial advice regarding Medicare and/or Medicaid and/or Veteran Benefits in the selecting of any specific insurance entity. Any state or federally mandated programs must be verified with the local state or federal government representatives.

The author's intent is to offer information on the healthcare system in a practical and useful way. The referrals to experts still require personal research in deciding the best tools and resources to select for any individual and personal situation.

The author assumes no personal or financial liability for any choices that may be decided upon after reading this information.

In order to protect the privacy of those mentioned in this book, names and certain identifying characteristics of patient situation and stories have been changed. Additionally, all stories were written following HIPPA (Health Portability Act of 1996) compliance guidelines.

Karyn Rizzo, Author, Patient Advocate, Consultant
ELITE Marketing & Consulting

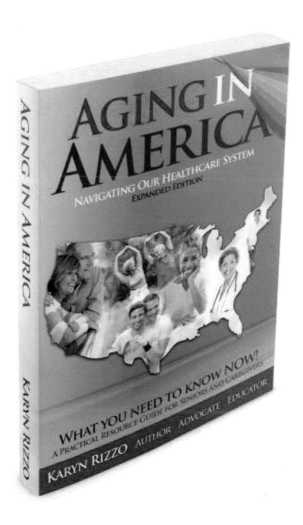

Contents

Contents Continued

PREFACE

The decision to write this handbook came after 20 years of working in the healthcare industry, in physician administration, hospitals and long term care nursing centers.

In that time, I witnessed a lot of sad situations happen to a variety of different patients. I could see the struggle that caregivers experienced to make the best decisions for their loved ones, in spite of so much confusing directions by their healthcare providers.

My hope is that this handbook can help older adults and their caregivers navigate our healthcare system with a better peace of mind.

After working with a variety of patients, physicians, hospital social workers, and insurance companies, I decided to use my knowledge to help more families have the needed information to understand our very complex healthcare system.

Daily I've witnessed the confusion that caregivers go through while trying to make the best medical decision for their loved ones. I've seen the agony and frustration experienced by patients trying to get accurate medical information, sometimes to no avail.

Since healthcare in America has become a very complicated maze, and is <u>**BUSINESS BASED**</u>, it can be very difficult to navigate the options and settings offered.

Furthermore, as each healthcare entity has a different financial agenda, with the common goal being to make a profit, knowing what the agenda is will ensure that you are truly making decisions that benefit you or your loved one, and not just becoming a number.

The helpful tips outlined will help you or a loved one navigate our healthcare system, and survive the "BUSINESS" of Aging in America.

INTRODUCTION

Aging in America may seem confusing to many elder patients and their caregivers. Trying to get straight, direct and honest answers can be difficult to come by.

WHY?

Simply put, it is because our healthcare system in America is a business and all businesses are trying to make a profit.

Therefore, many of the medical professionals and entities we trust have a financial agenda. Numbers not patients, bring profits. So when you know that you are a number, you can better understand why you are being directed in a certain direction.

I've seen older adults and their caregivers go through extreme anxiety due to the choices offered to them by their physicians, hospitals, and insurance companies.

Many times these patients do not even know they have other alternatives than the options they are being given. Therefore, many people suffer physical and financial consequences that could have been avoided.

Unfortunately, elderly people who have no one to protect them suffer even greater injustices. I could give countless examples that have broken my heart over the years, however, prefer to give information to protect others from harm.

The **INSIDER INFORMATION** provided here is to help you avoid the financial agendas of providers that may

14

unintentionally or intentionally cause harm to you or your loved one.

If you know *WHY* you're being directed in one direction over another, or understand why you're not being given some choices at all, hopefully it can help to make better decisions for you or your loved one.
Many times I hear the same question from patients and their caregivers:

Why did one provider only give me certain options?

Why did one provider make one recommendation and another one a completely different one?

The Insider information given here can help provide accurate and relevant information on the ever changing healthcare options and programs available to patients.

This handbook is intended to help elders and caregivers successfully navigate the complex maze of Aging in America.

STATISTICS ON AGING

- **70% of people 65 years young and older will need long term care**

- **77 million people born between 1946 and 1964, which is defined as the Baby Boom era (US Census)**

- **The senior age group (65 yrs. and up) is now, for the first time, the largest in terms of size and percent of population in the US**

- **Baby Boomers make up 35% of the American Adult population**

- **Life expectancy is inching closer to 100 years of age**

  2012 National Average Long Term Costs Are*:

- **$81,000 per year private room nursing home**

- **$73,000 per year semi-private room nursing home**

- **$40,000 per year Assisted Living**

- **$61 per day Adult Day Care Health Center**

- **$19 per hour Home Health Aide (non Medicare)**

- **$18 per hour Homemaker Services**

Since Americans are living longer, and have more healthcare choices than in the past, this book is meant to give a helpful overview of the key elements that can impact an aging person and their caregiver's experiences.

*Costs are according to the 2012 Genworth Financial Cost of Care Survey

CHAPTER 1

CHOOSING THE BEST PRIMARY CARE PHYSICIAN

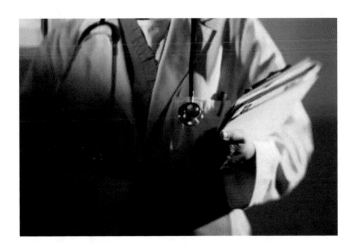

The Pilot of your Healthcare Journey!

CHOOSING A PRIMARY CARE PHYSICIAN

Why start with choosing a primary care physician?

Simply put, a primary care physician is the pilot of each person's healthcare journey.

Many elderly people choose a physician, or are assigned one by an insurance company, when relatively healthy, or for a temporary medical condition.

The physician may have been recommended by a friend, or have been assigned by an insurance company, and many have not evaluated the doctor to make sure they have the best one possible.

For many of them their doctor can become a part of their entire life, and very much like a member of the family, and by the time the senior is now aging, their primary physician is also.

Many older physicians do *NOT* still have active hospital privileges and some are not always up to date with the newest and best practices in medicine.

Why is this so important?

Once a senior has developed certain chronic medical conditions, such as high blood pressure, diabetes, chronic heart failure, or other conditions that require prescription management, this is where a physician that hasn't kept up with the latest information may be recommending outdated drugs or treatments, and may not be aware of the most current medication interactions and procedures.

Most often, a senior may have a loyalty to their physician, even if they aren't feeling better, due to the span of history they share. However, in the case of a medical emergency requiring a hospital or rehabilitation stay, this loyalty towards their doctor will not serve them well.

Unless a person has a lot of health issues, many only see their primary care physician a few times of year at best, and for a few brief minutes, if at all.

In the event of a sudden medical emergency or accident, the primary care physician becomes the **MOST** important person in a hospital setting. Therefore, choosing a primary care physician that is not only competent and well trained, can and will drastically affect the future choices and options a person will have available.

Since most humans are instilled with instincts that we will all live forever and never get ill, we usually don't think about the doctor we've chosen until we need them. And then we definitely will rely upon them!

Your primary care physician, who is the ultimate manager of your health journey, is the one that will be helping you decide what medications are needed, and in the event of a hospital stay will be the key person directing you or a loved one's recovery.

A primary care physician can become a friend,   concerned for your overall wellness, however **SHOULD** also be someone you can rely upon in the event of an unforeseen major illness, or medical emergency.

This choice is so crucial because it's important that the physician you've chosen is in agreement with your wishes, and up to date on all the latest medical advances.

Some have found out only **AFTER** they get taken to the hospital that their doctor does not have hospital privileges at all, or may not even be allowed at the hospital of their choice. Then they are even more surprised to find out that their care decisions are now being assigned to a virtual stranger.

So if a senior is attached to a physician that does **NOT** have hospital privileges, what can be done?

I've always recommended keeping the older doctor as a friend, invite them over for the holidays if you like, however, interview and select a _Board Certified_ Physician with **ACTIVE HOSPITAL PRIVELEGES** that can manage the aging loved ones ever changing medical needs.

Furthermore, most primary care physicians have alliances they make with specific hospitals, hospitalist physicians, rehabilitation centers, home health agencies, and Medicare and Medicaid replacement Insurance companies.

Why do they form these alliances?

Most physicians choose to align themselves with quality care organizations to protect them from malpractice claims and a damaging reputation.

However, for some physicians, due to the shrinking pay and rising operational expenses are influenced to make some decisions for their patients based on the money their alliances will pay them.

Due to the challenges of making money as a physician, many doctors have changed their practices to only treat patients on an outpatient basis, in their offices, while others have decided on only having a hospital based practice. Some doctors have chosen a hybrid method, in which they treat their patients in an outpatient setting but also follow them to the local hospitals and rehabilitation centers.

Across the nation, physicians are dealing with shrinking reimbursements from insurance companies, higher malpractice insurance costs and the daily challenges of running an office with ever increasing overhead.

Also, the physicians who DO take care of their patients while in a Hospital and/or Skilled Nursing and Rehab Centers like to have most of their patients in a convenient area, to maximize their very limited time.

Therefore, due to the shrinking income they're struggling with, these alliances pay their physicians as a medical director a monthly stipend or bonus, which can benefit as extra income for their practice. This may be a key factor as to WHY a physician is making a REFERRAL to a certain home care agency, hospital or rehabilitation center.

Usually a medical directorship or advisory position can pay a physician from $500.00 to $15000.00 per month, per entity

(Hospital, Skilled Nursing Center, and Home Health Agency) depending on the area in the country. Therefore, on a yearly basis this income collectively becomes a huge asset.

Contrary to what most people may stereotypically assume, not all physicians are rich, and some have enormous debt loads. Therefore, these additional incomes are something that they vehemently protect.

For instance, if a rehab center is looking at hiring a different Medical Director, to preserve this income, a doctor will be more feverishly looking for one of their patients to admit there, to reaffirm their worth, and preserve their job and income with that rehab center.

Also, some physicians have become contracted providers with Medicare and Medicaid Advantage Plans (HMO's), and receive money for their patient office visits, as well as monthly amounts per patient they have with the HMO Insurance Company, and those payments per patient payment can range from $5.00 to $30.00 or more, per patient /per month, which is commonly known as a monthly capped amount. They receive this monthly patient capped income from the Insurance companies, regardless if they've seen any of these patients that are members of the insurance company during the month, or NOT.

These Insurance Companies, who accept federal Medicare money and state Medicaid money are trying to maximize their profits, i.e. make their business profitable. Therefore, they may require certain services and specialties to be authorized, and impose limitations on the physicians as to what they are allowed to offer their patients, *and in some cases, despite what a patient's medical condition requires.*

Thus, many physicians struggle as they try to manage their patient's wellness and conditions within the limitations imposed upon them by the various

Insurance companies they are working with. At times this develops into situations where they are not able to practice medicine in the way that they've been trained and know to be more accurate.

For example, some Insurance contracts penalize a physician financially when they order certain costly tests, specialist consultations, rehab or home health services, and/or simply deny authorization for some or all of these services.

At times, when a physician wants their patients to have medical assistance in the home, an expensive medication, a specialty test or some other service or procedure that can make a difference in their health, they are simply not allowed to order these services.

What is maddening is that many of these are services and entitlements allowed under straight Medicare or Medicaid.

Our Federal Government actually give an incentive to these insurance companies to manage the distribution of benefits to the recipients entitled, but sadly, many find very legal and ingenious ways to avoid allowing and authorizing what they are required to do. With minimal oversight from the government, the Insurance companies have been able to get away with NOT providing members what their physician know they need.

Many times a physician's referrals can have financial consequences for them, and can influence the referrals they make. All physicians take an oath to "cause no harm," however, may struggle with their oath and the reality of making a profitable living at the same time.

Simply put, physicians are running a *BUSINESS* as well.

Therefore, the options that will be offered a patient while in the community or in the event of a hospital stay are always directed by the primary care physician, as long as they have *ACTIVE* hospital privileges.

If a primary care physician does <u>*NOT*</u> have hospital privileges, then a hospitalist physician will assume this role during the hospital stay. This virtual stranger will now be calling all the shots during the entire hospital stay, without having a previous understanding of the patient's medical history.

Hospitalist physicians can be either an independent physician that accepts patients whose physicians don't round in hospitals, or be employed by the hospital primarily and do not have any community offices.

While in the hospital, a primary care physician or hospitalist physician will be making medical decisions such as what tests, medications, specialty consultations, are needed.

This is where the alliances come into the picture. If the physician taking care of a patient in the hospital is the Medical Director of a certain skilled nursing center, they usually try to direct to those centers they work with.

HOPEFULLY, it's one preferred and is convenient to your support system.

Similarly, they usually follow suit if the patient is being discharged home, and will write an order for the company they work with, or is paying them a monthly stipend.

If there is a Commercial Insurance, Medicare or Medicaid replacement HMO, the options become even more limited. The influence of Medicare Advantage Plans will be covered in subsequent chapters.

Since a primary care physician is so crucial to anyone's future wellness, how can the best one be chosen?

There are many ways to obtain the best recommendations. Word of mouth is always an excellent way, however, the best recommendations come from someone who works in healthcare. Many healthcare employees have learned which physicians are the most ethical, and which may be best suited for someone's personal preferences (man, woman, nationality, etc.) and Insurance company.

Many have learned from some of their neighbors and friends experiences which ones are of a higher expertise and integrity. Most hospitals, senior centers and assisted living communities sometimes offer lectures and an opportunity to meet the physicians personally. At these sessions a potential patient has the opportunity to know that physician, and ask questions without having to set an appointment in their office.

With the influence of the internet, there are many different internet sites that grade and judge the quality of all local physicians, and include any pending malpractice claims against them.

This decision is so important to anyone's future health choices that a checklist is included to best judge weather a physician would be the best for you or a loved one, and be willing to work in harmony with your wishes.

Because you usually only have a very short time during an appointment to discuss specifics with any physician, a lot of the needed information can be gathered by looking around the office or asking the staff.

Additionally, most local hospitals have websites that list the physicians that have privileges with them, including their specialties, training, and usually a picture.

USEFUL TIPS

1. Do your research. Investigate a doctor you may be interested in online, and through word of mouth **BEFORE** you set an appointment. Ask if they are board certified and in what specialties (Board Certified physicians have additional training and testing).

2. <u>**INTERVIEW THE PHYSICIAN** (see Physician Interview form)</u> Find out what Hospitals, Nursing centers and Home Health agencies they primarily work with.

3. Do your research on the hospital and Rehab & nursing centers, and home health agencies online. Every state has an organization that survey these centers and agencies to judge what, if any, deficiencies they have.

4. Visit the hospitals and skilled nursing centers that **THIS PHYSICIAN** is primarily affiliated with.

5. Look very carefully at the brochures that are in your Drs. waiting room, as this is a clue to observe if your doctor has a few alliances, or "plays the Medical Director game", with many companies. This may become important as it may affect referrals to affiliates later on when needed.

6. It's also critical to know how many Medicare and Medicaid HMO's they are promoting, which again will limit your choices in the event of an emergency.

7. If the physician is owned by any Medicare Advantage Plan Insurance Companies, they may have an Insurance case manager that all authorizations go through.
8. It's also good to know if the physician practice is owned by any Hospitals. Hospitals have been purchasing some physician offices as well, and hopefully it is a hospital that you like, as you will be directed there, and to any other services they offer.

Make sure to bring a current medication listing including vitamin supplements that are being taken to save the physician's time.

Write down any specific questions about your health you may have for the physician in advance.

When a physician is owned by an Insurance company, sometimes, they are not at liberty at times to order certain tests or services their patients need as the insurance company must require prior approval.

When a Hospital owns a Dr.'s practice, the physician is not usually at liberty to make recommendations to any Hospital, Skilled Nursing center, or ancillary service other than the ones the Hospital owns.

There have been many cases where a physician, especially the ones owned by an Insurance company, may try to convince a patient that they don't need what the rest of the healthcare providers are saying they do.

For example, a physician once told a 66 year old woman that had just had a hip surgery that she didn't require physical therapy at a rehab center because she smoked and instead should just call in Hospice. Thankfully, the family was educated about their rights and the physician was forced to order and authorize the services she needed.

Her Medicare Advantage Plan's Case Manager was not happy. The Physician complained to my Administrator at the time about me because I informed the family of their rights to an appeal.

Sadly, these cases are not isolated and many seniors and families have found out while in the midst of a crisis that their physician was not the best choice for them.

If you don't feel comfortable with your primary care physician for any reason you should continue your search.

What is chiefly important is that whomever is chosen will have your best interests at heart and not their own pocketbook.

If your Medicare Advantage Plan has assigned a doctor that makes you uncomfortable for any reason, call the customer service line immediately, as they can usually offer to assign another doctor.

PHYSICIAN INTERVIEW FORM
(Ask the Staff for Answers)

What is the average age of his/her patient practice?

_____

What Hospital (s) do they admit to mostly? If they don't have hospital privileges, which Dr. (s) do they refer to, and what hospital do they work out of?

_____

What Skilled Nursing & Rehab Centers / "Nursing Homes" do they refer to? _____

Are they Medical Director / Adviser of any of them?

_____

What Home Health Agencies does he/she work with, and are they Director of any? _____

Is he/she Board Certified? Do they have Specialty training?

_____

Are they open to natural and alternative methods of treatments? _____

Are they part of any Medicare / Medicaid Advantage Plans / HMO? _____

Are the majority of their patients on Original Medicare or Medicare Advantage Plans? _____

Is the practice owned by a Hospital and/or Independent Physician Association (IPA)? _____

Many have found out the hard way that the hospital, skilled nursing centers, and home care agencies their primary care physician has referred them to, is substandard. Selecting the best partner for your healthcare journey can be done by researching physicians and their affiliations **CAREFULLY**.

For example, if a Dr. does a lot of clinical drug trials, which they get paid for by the pharmaceutical companies, may be prescribing more medications than needed. Also, some physicians, especially the ones that are **NOT** board certified have been known to overmedicate their patients, and/or prescribe outdated medications, which can lead to many unpleasant complications and side effects.

In one case, if a primary care physician who is the Medical director of a respiratory hospital, has consistently directed patients there, even if it may **NOT** be medically necessary, and especially when the census or patient occupancy is low.

In addition, there are certain times of the year when hospitals and skilled nursing centers have more open beds. This is the time when you or a loved one may be directed to a certain place, even if it's not medically necessary, or the recovery care could be handled at home.

In another case, a nursing home resident whose family lived out of town and went to the hospital to be treated for pneumonia. Because the census (occupancy rate) was low at his primary care physician's respiratory hospital affiliate which he was the medical director of, the patient was sent to that hospital, even though he did not meet the criteria, and his needs could easily be met at his nursing home, which had become his long term home.

Another example of how a physician can control what type of care you receive is evidenced by one physician whose husband is a Gastroenterologist and almost all of this doctor's nursing home residents get a standard order for a GI consult, by her husband, when they are admitted to the hospital. This is to see if they need a feeding tube in their stomach, whether they can swallow or not. A feeding tube, or peg tube are generally used to feed a patient when they cannot swallow any longer on their own. It is known by the hospital staff that this physician is helping her husband pay for their lifestyle by the choice of her recommendations for her nursing home patients, EVERY ONE.

In one case, her patient passed EVERY swallow test, and this physician was still insisting that the patient receive a feeding tube. Luckily, the hospital staff and family intervened so that this sweet senior who loved her sweets would not lose access to them.

GOOD MEDICAL MANAGEMENT STORY

Joan, 77 years young, had been very active, driving, involved in her church prior to a hospital stay, where she was assigned to an older hospitalist physician. He prescribed 3 additional medications and sent her home with Hospice Home Health. (Hospice in some areas functions as any other Medicare Home Health Agency billing Medicare).

Her conditioned worsened at home, and many at her church thought she was dying due to "Hospice" being called in.

Her Nurse and I case managed the medication situation and decided we needed to get a better physician consultation.

We called in a board certified Geriatrician, who made a house call. Two of her medications were contraindicated, or working against each other, so he changed her medications and within 2 days she was participating in therapy and on her way to a full recovery.

This demonstrated both the risk of getting admitted to a hospitalist that may work for the hospital, or simply not be up to date with medication best practices and current training.

There are seasonal changes that can affect how a physician directs their patients as well. For some areas, the slow season in some places may be during the summer, which means the physicians are under more pressure than usual from their affiliates to send them business, or patients. Thus, if you observe that the hospital you or your loved one is in seems highly quiet, it could be that they are having a slow time of the year for them. Be even more vigilant that the direction you or your loved one is sent are in direct harmony with your wishes.

As previously discussed, when a physician is the Medical Director of a Rehab center, these entities sometimes pay them thousands of dollars monthly, and expect the doctor to keep them busy with their patients. So during the slow times of the year, these doctors are under even more pressure to deliver patients to them, and that could end up being you or your loved one, despite your objections.

*** If you ever find yourself in this situation, ask to speak
with a social worker or case manager that works for the
hospital, as they can become an advocate for you or your
loved one's behalf. ***

Board Certified physicians are especially careful to align
themselves with the providers known for giving the highest
quality of care and with better reviews from the state
agencies. They not only have their medical license and
board status to protect, but also run the risk of more
malpractice claims when choosing providers to align their
practice with.

Older physicians that a senior may have had for many years,
and loves, may not be the best choice to manage them in a
hospital setting, if that becomes necessary. Therefore, the
best recommendation for a high quality ethical physician is
one that is Board Certified, has a lower percentage of
Managed Care Insurance companies that they contract with,
and is trained at handling patients during a hospital stay, or
has Board Certified hospitalists that they refer to.

With some research, and careful conversation, you can be
certain that your medical care is in the best of hands if a
hospital stay or more complex medical care is necessary.

The websites listed below can give a lot of useful information on a physician you may be considering or assigned to:

www.healthgrades.com   Healthgrades

www.ratemds.com   Rate MD's

www.vitals.com   Vitals

www.informedpatient.org   Informed Patient

www.hca.com   HCA

www.baycare.org   BayCare

www.va.gov   Veteran Administration

www.wellness.com   Wellness

CHAPTER 2

SELECTING INDEPENDENT & ASSISTED LIVING CENTERS

BEFORE THERE IS A NEED

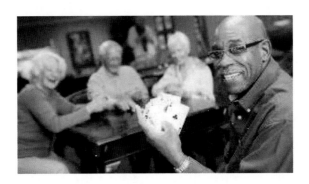

Tips for choosing long term care housing!

Fact: Some Seniors live 3-5 years longer when living in a long term care setting.

Although most seniors as they are aging are convinced that they will retire and die at home, and may say, "I'm only leaving my home feet first". This is simply a denial of the mind, as most people do not have this experience in their golden years.

Many people do not want to be reminded that they are aging, and simply avoid doing any preventative research that can have a huge impact on their future lives. Some very practical seniors have decided voluntarily to make their preparations on their own. To them ~ I say – Bravo!

The statistics show that 70 % of Americans will require help with the activities of daily living (ADL's) at some future point in time. There are six basic ADLs: eating, bathing, dressing, toileting, transferring (walking) and continence.

When a family accepts that their loved one will need additional help at some future point in the future, most likely in a healthcare center, it becomes reasonable to begin touring centers to be in a position to choose the best one.

Studies have shown seniors that have chosen a healthcare center for themselves, either prior to a need or during, have a much better transition emotionally, a lower anxiety rate and an extended life expectancy of an additional 3-5 years.

Some seniors have the means and desire to stay at home with private duty caregivers or a relative, but with the decline in the market recently, many seniors that had this as their main plan, suddenly may need to make adjustments.

Touring these centers can assist the hospital or rehabilitation center staff, and/or your primary care physician in making sure your choices are honored in the event they are needed. Many healthcare living centers offer parties and lunches at no charge to help introduce their community to the public.

For instance, some whom are living in their home and declining, may have family arrive from out of town on a visit, who suddenly realize how care they actually now require, and begin the process of choosing a center for them, usually in panic mode, and much against their will.

Resulting in a much more difficult transition, given the personalities involved, than if a senior is able to choose for themselves an Independent, Assisted Living or Skilled Nursing Center.

With so many different types of healthcare settings available, let's examine the variety of options with the objective to search more efficiently.

There are often local counties that have different senior living magazines and websites featuring many of these communities that are available, and usually at no charge.

Many seniors believe that the only choice they have is home or a "nursing home", however, there are so many more options for senior living than ever in our nation's history.

INDEPENDENT LIVING CENTERS & SENIOR APARTMENT LIVING

These communities require that their residents be able to perform most of the activities of daily living independently and without assistance.

Activities of daily living are eating, bathing, dressing, toileting, transferring (walking) and continence.

These very basic mandatory requirements are crucial to a senior being able to live safely in these communities. Some residents also still own and drive a car in senior apartment living and independent communities. Most are also "pet friendly" as long as the pet is a certain size and up to date with vaccination records. Many communities do have a pound restriction, ranging from 15 to 50 pounds.

The monthly rent usually includes meals, housekeeping, local transportation and social activities. Most independent living centers also have some nursing services or a home health agency available if medications need to be managed. Senior apartment staff may offer connections to outside resources when more care is needed.

Most of these centers try to attract very healthy and active seniors without the need for a cane or walker to get around. Choosing this type of community early is recommended as this can help maintain a senior's independence and activity level.

Independent Living Centers or Senior Apartments offer very minimal assistance.

Most of these communities charge rent monthly, with an annual contract. The charges will vary based on location, and the amenities offered. The benefits to the residents are that they usually have access to transportation, housekeeping and social activities.

Also, there are many Continuing Care Retirement communities that offer the same services, some on a month to month rental basis, and others with a "buy in" option.

There are also low income properties that offer this style of living and only charge a percentage of the senior's social security income, and /or assets, which can be a great option, especially if the only income is social security or a small pension.

ASSISTED LIVING CENTERS

These centers provide much more assistance with the activities of daily living than Independent living centers or senior apartment communities. They do require that the resident be able to transfer with supervision only, depending on the type of license they have, and the licensing requirements of the state they are located in.

In some states, there are advanced assisted living licenses that allow them to perform more assistance, such as a "limited nursing" or "extended congregate care" licenses. These licenses allow them to manage diabetes, and provide more assistance with a resident's activities of daily living.

Many Assisted living centers also offer day care usually costing around $50 – $150.00 per day which is a nice way for a senior to get familiar with their services and community.

Some also offer short term respite stays, which is another way of exposing a senior to the center without actually having to move in.

The cost for assisted living centers vary based on the area and the amenities they offer.

Many are pet friendly, and will allow a dog or cat to be less than 25 to 35 pounds. Of course, they usually require that the resident be able to care for their pet, however, some places offer pet care at a nominal charge.

Some states offer assistance paying for assisted living care under their Medicaid program. We'll cover the Medicaid coverage in a later chapter.

Shopping for Assisted Living is much like shopping for a car, do so late in the month, if possible and feel free to negotiate the monthly rate. Also, it's helpful to make the rate good for a year to be sure that there are no unexpected rent hikes later.

MEMORY CARE ASSISTED LIVING CENTERS

Many assisted living centers have an area that is secured and have activity programs to assist residents with the symptoms of Alzheimer's disease or dementia. The requirements for these centers are usually the same as assisted living with the key difference that the residents usually are at risk of elopement requiring a secured environment for their safety.

Memory Care Assisted Living Centers offer more engagement programs, and some have been built in accordance with new research on the managing symptoms and reality that a dementia patient experience.

These newer *Memory Care Living Centers* are a great alternative to mainstream assisted living centers, however, can be somewhat more expensive.

The staff are usually specifically selected and trained to manage the behaviors that an aging dementia person experiences, such as sun downing and other behaviors.

Like choosing any assisted living community, research on recent state surveys, corporation ownership, and the longevity of the staff are key areas to take notice of.

The local Alzheimer's Association chapter offer support groups that can assist in referring caregivers to local facilities that offer this type of assisted living, either on a short respite or permanent basis.

The websites listed below can help you to find a local chapter.

www.alzfdn.org   Alzheimer's Association

www.alfa.org   Assisted Living Federation of America

www.caring.com/assisted-living Caring

www.healthcarefinder.gov Healthcare Finder

CONTINUING CARE RETIREMENT COMMUNITIES (CCRC)

This is a community that offers all levels of care, Independent, Assisted Living and Skilled Nursing and Rehabilitation center. They are either a monthly private pay fee or a buy in community, and in some cases, a combination of both.

The advantage some find in these communities is that a resident can transition to the next care level as their healthcare needs increase.

The warning for a "buy in" communities are that some seniors have bought into them, at a substantial fee, and have not been pleased with the services, or found that they never needed the amount of care levels they had paid for.

Most Independent and Assisted Living centers are on a month to month rental basis, especially due to the uncertain nature of a seniors future health needs. The freedom and flexibility of a monthly rent system can be appealing to many seniors as they have the ability to change their surroundings if they become unpleased with the care or require more help.

WE'VE CHOSEN A CENTER, HOW DO I GET MY LOVED ONE TO AGREE TO MOVE IN?

To start, many seniors that need more care than they can have or afford at home refuse to accept any changes in their environment. Some seniors are in denial of their own care needs, forcing the adult child to become the parent. You wouldn't allow a child to determine their care needs and although it's very difficult to do, an unreasonable senior, especially with any kind of safety issues, should not be making these decisions either.

One way to get a senior to try a long term care center is to go on vacation, and have them stay at a center on a short term / respite basis. It sounds selfish, but this is one way to allow them to try an active retirement center without forcing an actual move. Most places offer a respite package, and this can be either a weekend or longer. Many times when a senior is moving into a long term care setting, their house may need repair. It's always recommended to tent the house, renovate bathrooms or kitchens if needed, to motivate them to stay at a preferred center, on a trial basis.

Most seniors comment after moving into a center they now realize that they should have done this a long time prior, and have reported they feel more energetic than before. The "tough love" approach, while not easy, is still in their best interests.

Sometimes involving a Geriatric Case Manager, Physician, Religious Leader, or Social Worker can assist in this transition process for no cost or very minimal charges.

The benefits of nutrition, socialization and interaction with peers cannot be underestimated. The quality of life that a resident of a nice senior living center is most often much more than they were able to receive at home, in some cases, watching television and eating poorly.

www.caremanager.org National Association of Professional Geriatric Care Managers

FINDING & PAYING FOR LONG TERM CARE

Long term care is on the minds of many people, regardless of their current health situation. Deciding what direction to go when choosing long term care providers can be very confusing. Now that more people are living longer, we're all facing decisions that most of us never have had to choose in the past.

What programs are available to help pay for long term care? In a nutshell, unless you were able to benefit from a long term care policy purchased early in life, then the National and State programs are what are able to pay for care. Sadly, in lieu of a long term care insurance policy, private savings and money that has been saved will be needed for retirement care.

Once a person is receiving disability benefits, or 65 years and older, Medicare can then offer Skilled Nursing, Physical, Occupational and Speech Therapies in wherever a person call home. This does need to be ordered by a primary care physician, and is one way to receive the additional care needed at no charge.

For those that have served in the Military, and have been honorably discharged, there are some low to no cost benefits and programs available. The Aid & Attendance benefit and many other benefits may cover private duty homecare, and assisted living when needed.

There is an asset cap to these programs; however, if a veteran or spouse is depending on low to little assets, the County Veteran Service Offices can help apply for benefits at no charge. In Pinellas County, simply contact Pinellas County Veteran Services at (727) 582-7828 for FREE assistance.

One can be found at the **NATIONAL ASSOCIATION OF COUNTY VETERAN SERVICE OFFICERS** at http://nacvso.org/find-a-service-officer/ .

To find a low costing service to help with the application of benefits, contact Elder Veterans Legal Aid Group 800-878-2149 (Low Cost).

If there is over $80,000 in assets, contact an Elder Law Attorney that specializes in VA benefits to begin the application. To find an elder law attorney in your area, go to www.naela.com

For information on the VA Health System and to meet with a Benefits officer, go to www.VA.org.

APPLYING FOR SOCIAL SECURITY DISABILITY

To apply for Social Security Disability Application Online http://www.ssa.gov/disabilityssi/ There are four steps in the Online Disability Application Process: Provide Background Information, Provide Disability Information, Sign Medical Release, and Confirmation (Takes 2 hours).

Many states offer long term care through Medicaid and this can be an option for many needing private duty assistance in the home and/or Assisted Living. In some states a Personal Needs Trust can be established by an elder law attorney, thus qualifying for the Medicaid benefits to pay for needed care.

If a Medicare recipient is living strictly on their SSI or SSD income, they most likely qualify for Community Medicaid and other state programs. To apply for Medicaid, the application can begin online at www.medicaid.org (enter state).

Those that have purchased a long term care insurance or disability policy will be able to use that to pay for care and assistance when needed. For those that cannot or are unable to purchase a policy, the other government programs then become a much needed alternative.

When choosing what type of long term care setting is right for an older adult, many key items become important, such as what type of assistance is needed with Activities of Daily Living, Location, Longevity of the Team, and Overall Wellness of the current Residents.

Always tour, and meet with the center being considered to determine if it will be a good match to the older adult's needs.

BENEFITS OF SENIOR CARE LIVING

Many aging adults prefer to stay at home where they can enjoy a retirement filled with social, safe and healthy activities. It isn't surprising that 75% of older adults plan to live in their current homes for the rest of their lives, according to the 2015 United States of Aging Survey, a joint project of the National Association of Area Agencies on Aging, the National Council on Aging, and United Health Care.

However, that isn't always the reality or choice for every older adult.

According to the U.S. Bureau of the Census, slightly more than 5% of the 65 years plus population occupy nursing homes, congregate care, assisted living, and independent senior living.

Throughout the years, on many occasions residents have said "I wished I would have made the move here sooner!"

What they weren't expecting is that their quality of life had increased with socialization, exercise, nutrition, and mental stimulation.

Some benefits to making the move early mean that there are many more options to choose from, before health limitations may set arise. Also, some have actually found that by moving into senior living sooner they have been able to save more money than they had thought.

The key benefits to an older adult choosing and moving into senior living are in four key areas.

Save on Home Expenses

More than 70% of homeowners ages 50 to 64 were still paying their mortgages in 2010, according to the U.S. News & World Report. The expenses of owning a home, in particular an older one, includes updating, property taxes, utilities, and homeowners insurance that can add up to more than $6,000 per year for homeowners. Furthermore, as care needs increase, there is usually a need for grab bars in the showers, ramps, and more.

Senior living communities provide all of these services and allow for their residents to reserve their energy being spent in ways they prefer.

Save your Nutritional Health

Eating well is important for any age group, but as we age it becomes even more crucial to an older adult's health. Consistently, poor nutrition occurs in the older population, especially after the loss of a spouse. Carefully planned meals and nursing oversight can result in a healthier, longer life span.

Save on Housekeeping

Daily Chores can be hard work, and are often the cause for many home falls. Falls are the leading cause of death in older adults, and a retirement community offers these services to allow for more time in other activities.

Save your Social Fun

Although most aging adults desire active social lives, many may find that limited mobility and other medical issues prevent them from doing so. Many studies have shown a direct connection to the mood and outlook of an aging adult's life and their physical health. Living in a retirement community offers endless opportunities to develop close social friendships, and engage in hobbies, games, travel, and fun events.

Ultimately, each aging adult has the right to stay in any SAFE environment they call home, however, the benefits to living in retirement communities should not be overlooked. Personally, those who've chosen a place for themselves seem to have the highest satisfaction with their retirement activities and overall wellness.

To begin the search for the RIGHT retirement community, go to www.healthcarefinder.gov

CHAPTER 3

CHOOSING A REHABILITATION CENTER

Aka "A NURSING HOME"

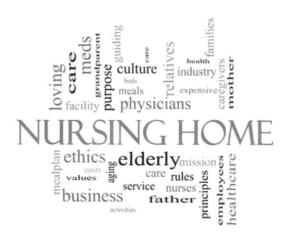

What to Look for when Touring Centers!

SKILLED NURSING & REHAB CENTERS aka "NURSING HOMES"

Skilled Nursing and Rehab Centers provide both short term rehabilitation, and long term custodial care. The short term rehabilitation includes physical, occupational, speech therapies, IV medications, wound care and much more.

The long term residents living in skilled nursing centers are usually residents that need assistance with most, if not ALL of their activities of daily living.

Most seniors that need short term rehab in a center do go back to their home, or to an independent or assisted living facility, depending on the care needs of the patient upon discharge.

Not all Skilled Nursing & Rehab centers are created equal, and it's important to tour and see the condition of the residents living there to make informed choices in advance.

The most urgent decision that causes a lot of stress on caregivers is when a loved one is in a hospital, and they're told that the doctors want their loved one to go to a Skilled Nursing & Rehab center. Sometimes they are being discharged and the hospital needs a decision NOW, or YESTERDAY.

The hospital staff will sometimes decide for the patient if a facility has not already been chosen.

Therefore, knowing in advance a place that is preferred, takes the urgent stress out of this type of situation.

How do you choose a place we wished we never would have had to?

Very Carefully!

Choosing a rehab center can be so important to a senior's future, it cannot be overstated. If a place causes them to be even further depressed or hopeless, it will most likely be the last place they live on earth.

If the center is known to have a high rate of discharging patients, they will most likely have a better experience, and be in a position to discharge sooner.

Also, notice how long the staff has been working together. The longer they have been working together, in most cases, the better chance of recovery and discharging home.

If there has been a lot of staff turnover, state deficiencies, and a **LOW CENSUS** (ask what the occupancy census is), that is a **BAD SIGN, RUN!**

The most important thing to look for when touring a rehabilitation and skilled nursing center is the condition of the residents, and the professionalism and kindness of the staff.

Every state has an inspecting agency and a website that can help find out what the most recent survey results were, as well as any penalties or fines. It's still best to tour personally as a lot of the information online can be quite out of date.

http://www.medicare.gov/nursinghomecompare

When touring skilled nursing centers, the touring form listed next can be most helpful.

All Skilled Nursing Centers should also have a copy available of their most recent state survey. Keep in mind that survey teams have to find some "tags" or areas to cite a facility on, however, if they are serious tags that endanger a patient's health or life, that can be a dangerous sign.

Furthermore, each center differs in the types of rehabilitation programs they offer and specialize in. For instance, there are some that are very good with younger psychiatric patients, and if a loved one does not suffer from those conditions, it would be best to keep looking. Usually, the doctors and hospital staff know which centers take what type of patient, insurance, etc. and can be a helpful resource when looking.

It's ok to ask a lot of questions, but more important to look at the current staff members, and patients that are currently there.

The attached Tip Sheet is to help you focus on the areas that can become crucially important after admission.

TIP SHEET "Nursing Homes"

What type of deficiencies did the center receive at their last state inspection? _____

How often is physical therapy provided? _____

What is the percentage of residents that are long term versus short term rehab? _____

What insurances does the center have contracts with?

_____

Does my physician have rounding privileges here?

_____

What is the staff to patient ratio (some states regulate this)?

_____

How many patients discharge home weekly? _____

What are the biggest complaints the residents in house have? _____

Can it pass the "SNF" / SNIFF Test?

_____

Aside from the "sniff test", meaning any smells of urine when entering, also note how the residents are dressed, and their overall appearance. Observe the staff, how attentive they are to the current resident's and their overall happiness with their job.

If possible, talk to some of the current residents and ask them about their day.

No matter how good a rating a center can have by the state rating agency, it only takes a change in management for that status to change, despite the ratings.

For instance, there was a 5 star rated facility that was put on a national focus list meaning they were being surveyed by state and federal inspections every 6 months due to their lack of compliance. So although they had in the past been a 5 star rated facility, that status had dropped drastically, yet the website (3 years old) continued listing them as a 5 star facility.

If your instincts are telling you that this isn't a good fit for you or your loved one, trust your instincts. Most staff would prefer not to admit someone against their wishes, as usually the transition is much more difficult for all concerned.

Furthermore, you would know best where your loved one will be most comfortable, and will need to visit the center regularly during their stay.

<u>HOW DO I MOVE A LOVED ONE OUT OF A CENTER IF A DIFFERENT ONE IS PREFERRED?</u>

So, let's say that the research has been done, and you or your loved one, want to move to a different center. How do you get them moved?

First, all of these centers with the exception of senior apartments and Independent living centers require a written physician's order of some kind. The form a physician has to fill out are state specific, however, the admissions department of every Assisted Living and Skilled Nursing and Rehab centers will know and have these forms.

The process usually starts with the center you prefer making a determination that your loved one has and/or, will be accepted. To allow the new center to do an evaluation simply let the Administrator or Social Service Director know that another center will be coming in to evaluate. Most centers will not accept a new resident sight unseen, unless they are coming from out of the area.

Once the new center has the required paperwork, transportation simply needs to be arranged. Most centers do NOT cover the cost of transportation, and neither Medicare nor Medicaid will pay for a "center to center" transfer.

If you or your loved one requires an ambulance, that can become quite costly. It's important to evaluate the care required, and count the cost.

Sometimes, attempting to reconcile with the current center can change you or your loved one's experience.

If you encounter any resistance from the current center regarding making a transfer or in resolving current care issues, you can also call in your local Ombudsman officer to try to mediate. Ombudsman is part of the National Long-Term Care Resource Center.

It's key to remember that some seniors are not going to be happy anywhere they are, sadly. If the care has suddenly changed for the worse, it's also good to find out if a new corporation has purchased them.

Most Assisted Living and Skilled Nursing Centers are owned by a handful of the same corporations. Moving your loved one from one healthcare center to a different one that is owned by the same company may not increase your loved one's experience.

Many of the reasons why care can change in an Assisted Living or Skilled Nursing and Rehab Center is directly linked to what they pay their nursing staff. If a new corporation has taken over that pays less than the current market rate, it can create a great degree of turnover, which also can result in the declining care.

Most importantly, it's important for families and extended families to have a strong presence in whatever center their loved one lives in to ensure the highest and best care.

If there is ever a disagreement between a Resident and the staff at a center, the local state authorities can be called, however, try to contact the Local Ombudsman Officer prior, to see if the issues can be resolved. If you or a loved one is staying long term than resolving care issues in the most diplomatic way possible is best for a patient depending on the care they need to receive.

202-332-2275   National Long Term Care Resource
                Center / Local Ombudsman

FACILITY LIVING SUMMARY

The more prepared for additional health care center needs, the better. Handling these choices before they're needed can make a senior's experience drastically better and even more so when they're involved in the decision making.

In some areas, there are companies that offer to serve as a liaison to assist families in making a choice in senior housing options. They usually offer this service at no charge to a senior or family, but may charge the facility a fee, such as one month's rent, depending on the state laws.

At times, if there are multiple family members that can't decide, these liaisons can serve as an unbiased voice to outline the pros and cons for each place.

Obviously, having a strong and regular visitation at any community will better ensure that a loved one gets the care they need.

To summarize, **RESEARCH, RESEARCH!**

CHAPTER 4

ESTABLISHING ADVANCE DIRECTIVES

<u>BEFORE NEEDED</u>

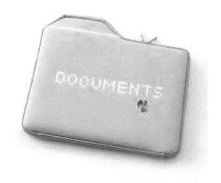

** Living Will*

** Do Not Resuscitate (DNR)*

** Healthcare Surrogate*

** Durable Power of Attorney (DPOA)*

WHAT ARE ADVANCED DIRECTIVES AND WHY ARE ESTABLISHING THEM SO IMPORTANT?

Advance Directives are your specific healthcare wishes put into writing in the event that you become unable to express your wishes for yourself. It explains to your loved ones and medical professionals exactly what medical measures you want taken, or NOT taken, in the case of an unexpected medical emergency or medical condition that causes you to be unable to speak for yourself.

Many believe that because they know what or how they would like to be medically treated, if the need arises, that those people closest to them will know as well.

How many times, perhaps watching a movie or witnessing a real life experience, we may think "I would scream if they put me through that"? Probably as often as we hear the evening news, or watch a medical show on television.

That's why having Advance Directives spelled out in writing is so very important. If your loved ones don't have your wishes in writing, they can't make sure that you are taken care of the way you would like.

Many have mistakenly thought that "my loved one knows what I would or would not want DONE to me," only to find out later that there are huge misunderstandings.

This situation happened to me personally. There was a very public medical case that drew nationwide attention that let me know that my healthcare proxy did not agree with my personal wishes, put in the same situation.

This very sad case had the media reporting the dispute in that the parents wanted their daughter to have a feeding tube in her stomach (peg tube), and her husband fighting against it.

This tragic and heartbreaking case brought to light that my own personal Healthcare proxy (my mother) needed to be changed.

It's a good idea after writing out Advance Directives to make sure they are discussed and understood by all involved. It's very important to make sure all clearly understand what certain medical phrases mean.

Many seniors have suffered in ways they did not want, simply because they never reduced their wishes in writing in a clear and easily understood way.

LIVING WILL

A living will is very different than a financial Will, which outlines the distribution of financial assets in the event of a death.

A Living Will outlines very specifically what conditions a person wants taken to preserve or not preserve their life. This is vital in communicating to the medical professionals about HOW and WHAT medical procedures are preferred in a medical emergency. The forms are listed at the websites below, and may be state specific.

This document makes a person really decide about what types of medical treatments they would want taken, one way or the other, and most importantly, makes it so that you or your loved one chooses, instead of the medical community, and helps medical professionals comply with personal wishes.

It's ok to add to a living will phrases like "no tubes", "hospice care welcome", "comfort measures only" for example.

The more specifics are on this document, the better.

DO NOT RESUSCITATE (DNR)

When a person is making decisions for their Living Will, most often a Do Not Resuscitate (DNR) form enters the discussion.

This is a document that states that in the event of a life threatening medical condition, the medical professionals are NOT to resuscitate the patient.

Until a patient is made a "Do Not Resuscitate" (DNR), they are a FULL CODE status, meaning the medical staff will use all available methods to resuscitate the patient. Thus, if a patient stops breathing, ALL methods will be used to save a life.

This may include having a tube down your throat or cracking open your chest to assist you in breathing.

This status at times creates confusion for many families. If someone has chosen to have a Do Not Resuscitate (DNR), it does NOT mean that the medical professionals no longer treat the patient medically. It simply means if they stop breathing, they will not be using EXTREME measures to resuscitate them. It does not mean 'DO NOT TREAT". There are still many treatment choices that will need to be made.

Such routine decisions can include treating infections, as simple as inserting a more permanent IV port, or as serious as deciding to have a more serious surgical procedure.

There are many hard decisions that have to be made at the end of a person's life and very careful and clear communication assists staff in making the best decision possible when these occasions arise.

This is why the person chosen to protect a person's healthcare choices is so important.

The person chosen to protect basic medical choices has to be the most reliable and ethical person possible.

The reason why that person is so important is covered in the later on in this book, and that is THE SECOND most important choice anyone can make.

HEALTH CARE PROXY / HEALTHCARE POWER OF ATTORNEY (POA)

Regardless of what state you live in, these are the two most common legal forms of designating a person to decide important medical and financial matters for you in the event you can't speak for yourself.

These forms can be the most difficult to decide. Healthcare Proxy is a form that gives a person power to decide healthcare decisions for you, and only healthcare decisions for you, and ONLY in the event the patient cannot speak for themselves.

Durable Power of Attorney is a legal document that gives someone power to utilize bank accounts to pay bills, execute important business decisions, and make healthcare decisions, in the event they cannot perform such tasks personally.

For instance, there may be a family member or close friend that may be trusted with financial decisions but not healthcare decisions, and vice-versa.

It's ideal to have a trusted family member be able to be Healthcare proxy and Durable Power of Attorney (DPOA) however, this is not always available or wise.

Because this person holds power over finances, and healthcare needs, this person needs to be chosen very carefully.

I've seen perfectly legal yet horrific things happen to people by their legal Durable Power of Attorney.

DURABLE POWER OF ATTORNEY (DPOA)

This form was established to assist families to conduct financial business for a loved one who may not be able to take care of things during a medical emergency.

*This person should be the **MOST TRUSTED AND FINANCIALLY STABLE FAMILY MEMBER OR LIFETIME FRIEND**.*

The enormous amount of power this person has, involving both healthcare and financial decisions, means that they need to be a very trustworthy person.

Some have abused this power to their own financial benefit, and at times to a senior's detriment.

Having a family member that is struggling financially is not a great choice for this role, as the temptation to take advantage may result in a senior not being taken care of.

It is very possible to have one trusted family member as the healthcare proxy, and another different family member as the Durable Power of Attorney. These forms on occasion may need to be changed, and should always be given to the person that's chosen for their records.

These forms should be easy to find, in the event of an unexpected medical emergency. These forms will also need to be given to any medical professionals in the event of an emergency.

BELOW ARE SOME SAMPLE WEBSITES FOR EACH STATE SPECIFIC FORM:

www.caringinfo.org

www.aarp.org

www.putitinwriting.org

www.edmedicinehealth.com

www.agingwithdignity.org

www.nlm.nih.gov/medlineplus/advanceddirectives.html

CHAPTER 5

FINANCIAL & HEALTHCARE PREFERENCES IN WRITING

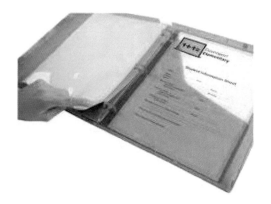

"The single biggest problem with communication is the illusion that it has taken place."

George Bernard Shaw

IMPORTANT PAPERS IN SEPARATE BINDER / FILE (EASY TO FIND)

Now that we know the different Advanced Directives and paperwork that can be crucial to a senior having their wishes upheld, we need to get a practical system that a family will need to have access to.

Since seniors are living longer, and there are so many more choices than in previous years, it's very important that all wishes are put in writing.

Also, it is extremely helpful if they are easily accessible for the family or support system.

Ideally, it's best to have 3 ring folder or binder with all of the most important documents readily available.

It should have all advanced directive documents, Healthcare Proxy, Durable Power of Attorney documents, a Do Not Resuscitate (if one is in place), as well as local banking contact information. If there is a family or Elder Law Attorney that has helped with these documents or financial affairs, their contact information should also be included.

If a financial will is in place, some seniors have their attorney hold on to it, or in a safety deposit box to avoid any family members fighting over belongings.

Many Husbands/ Fathers have always handled all the financial affairs, and unfortunately some wives have not had access to the specific finances. Subsequently, if the husband/father has a sudden medical condition that renders him unable to communicate these specifics, a 3 ring binder can help the family know how to conduct business on their behalf.

Many families have experienced many unnecessary bills because the family member that has become ill is unable to conduct business as usual, and no information has been shared with the family members.

Certain banks will not conduct business, even necessary business, with family members unless these legal documents are presented.

This suggestion may sound simplistic to families that have open communication and have an organized game plan in the event of an emergency. With so many families in the "sandwich situation" raising their own families and managing an aging parent, the time to get around to these very important papers can make life much simpler when they're needed. This can be very difficult if the aging parent is private about financial matters.

For families with estranged relationships that haven't been mended, the result can be even more severe for a senior.

When should these matters be setup for a senior? The answer comes down to their general health. There are healthy, active seniors that live to 90 plus years; however, they are the rarest of our population. If a senior has had multiple medical conditions at a young age or have experienced the following medical conditions: high blood pressure, high/low blood sugar, cardiac problems, obesity, arthritis, joint disease, kidney problems, cancer or any other major disease that requires medication, the time is <u>NOW</u>, or <u>YESTERDAY.</u>

<u>Checklist for Binder</u>

- ➢ Living Will
- ➢ Do Not Resuscitate
- ➢ Healthcare Proxy
- ➢ Durable Power of Attorney
- ➢ Financial Power of Attorney
- ➢ Bank Account Information
- ➢ Life Insurance Policies
- ➢ Family or Elder Law Attorney contact information
- ➢ ** Financial Will & Letter of Instruction ** (Attorney or Safe Deposit Box)

KEEP AN ENVELOPE TAPED TO THE REFRIDGERATOR WITH ALL HEALTHCARE DOCUMENTS & CURRENT MEDICATION LISTING

Emergency Medical Professionals are trained to look there in case of a medical emergency.

CHAPTER 6

ORIGINAL MEDICARE vs. MEDICARE ADVANTAGE PLAN

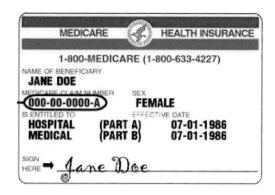

"Peace is the Result of retraining your mind to process life as it is, rather than you as you think it should be."

Dr. Wayne W. Dyer

ORIGINAL MEDICARE versus
MEDICARE ADVANTAGE PLAN "HMO"

While writing this chapter and waiting for my car to be fixed, I overheard an adult child and her aging mother discussing whether she should get on Original Medicare or a Medicare Advantage Plan when she turned 65 next month. Of course, I stopped to help them understand what factors are essential in making this decision.

Many people do not realize that in America medicine is **BIG BUSINESS, NOT A HUMAN SERVICE.** Many times people fight the idea of socialized medicine; however, the countries that have successfully established it, consider healthcare a human service. In those countries doctors are paid by preventative care percentages, and their citizens, for the most part, do receive what they need without going broke. Obviously, not all countries have mastered the kinks out of their healthcare systems, but America does remain one of the few countries where one major illness or hospital stay can deplete a person's savings and/or result in bankruptcy. The same principle applies to receiving Medicare benefits when eligible.

Thus, the decision to have Original Medicare or a Medicare Advantage Plan is a **BUSINESS ONE.** There are essential factors that need to be carefully considered when making this decision. First, let's understand how Medicare works.

MEDICARE is a federal health insurance program for eligible individuals. It has no spousal / dependent coverage and does **NOT** cover long term custodial care. It's administered by the Centers for Medicare & Medicaid Services (CMS).

ELIGIBILITY REQUIREMENTS: You must be a United States Citizen or legal, permanent resident of the United States for at least 5 continuous years prior to enrollment. You must be at least 65 years old or if under 65: receiving Social Security disability income for at least 24 months, or have End State Renal Disease (ESRD) or Amyotrophic Lateral Sclerosis (ALS) "Lou Gehrig's Disease".

ENROLLMENT is coordinated by the Social Security Administration (SSA), or Railroad Retirement Board (RRB).

➢ Initial Enrollment Period: 7 months prior to 65th Birth month.
➢ General Enrollment Period: January 1st through March 31st. Coverage starts July 1st.
➢ Annual Election Period a.k.a. "Fall Open Enrollment": October 15th through December 7th. Changes effective January 1st. For those already in Medicare, join or switch Medicare Advantage Plans, return to Original Medicare, or add, drop of switch Medicare Prescription drug plans.
➢ Special Enrollment Periods: Original Medicare – working past age 65 with Employer Group, moving out of plan's coverage area, Involuntary loss of coverage, Qualify for Medicaid Assistance.
➢ Medicare Advantage Disenrollment Period:
➢ January 1st through February 14th. Disenroll from any Medicare Advantage Plan and return to Original Medicare with optional standalone drug coverage.

<u>WHAT ARE MY MEDICARE CHOICES?</u>

There are two main ways to get Medicare Coverage: Original Medicare or a Medicare Advantage Plan.

Use these steps to help decide on a coverage plan: Start

Step 1: Decide how you want to get your coverage.

Original Medicare   or   Medicare Advantage
Part C "HMO/PPO"

Part A – Hospital Insurance
Part B – Medical Insurance   Part A, B & usually D

Step 2: Decide if you need to add drug coverage.

Part D – Prescription Plan   Included in most
plans

Step 3: Add supplemental coverage?

**Medicare Supplemental
(MEDIGAP POLICY)**

**Cannot buy a
Supplemental
Insurance Policy**

ORIGINAL MEDICARE: *PARTS A & B*
"Fee for Service"

➢ Can go to any provider that accepts Medicare (usually anywhere).

➢ No authorization required for any Inpatient or Outpatient Care.

❖ Part A – covers Inpatient Hospital Care, Blood, Skilled Nursing Care, Home Health Services, and Hospice Care. 80 – 100% medically necessary services covered.

❖ Part B – covers Doctors Services, Outpatient Medicare, Durable Medical Equipment, Preventative Services. 20% co-payment due on most services.

❖ Does not cover Vision, hearing, dental, travel coverage, private duty nursing, or long term custodial care.

ORIGINAL MEDICARE COSTS *
Part A

➢ **2016 Premium: Free for most (need 40 work credits)**

➢ **2016 Hospital Deductible $1288.00**

Part B
➢ **2016 Premium Cost: $104.90**
➢ **2016 Annual Deductible: $166.00**

High Earners Part B Premiums
➢ **Single Earners ($85000 - $107,000) $146.90**
➢ **Single Earners (over $214,000) $335.70**

*Please refer to www.medicare.gov and www.cms.gov for annual changes in pricing. (2016 Medicare Costs)

<u>MEDICARE SUPPLEMENTAL/ "Medigap"</u>

➢ Pays for payment gaps in Original Medicare (co-pays etc.)
➢ Provided by Independent Health Insurance Companies (costs vary).
➢ All benefits have to be the exact same, regardless of differing costs (shop diligently)
➢ Enrollment Period: Up to 6 months following Medicare Part A & B.

MEDICARE ADVANTAGE PLANS
"HMO /Managed Care"

➢ Part A & B Services covered (co-payments may apply).
➢ May reimburse for part or all of Part B premiums.
➢ May include Prescription Drug Coverage.

➢ May include Vision, hearing, and dental, travel etc.

❖ Must use in network Primary Care Physician and providers.
❖ May charge high daily Co-Payments for hospital, Skilled Nursing Centers, and some specialty treatments and surgeries.
❖ Requires authorization by Insurance Case Manager or Primary Care Physician for specialty physicians.

❖ Requires authorization for home health services.
❖ 1 year mandatory trial period. (May disenroll if relocating).

Enrollment Period:
October 15th – December 7th

Disenrollment Period:
January 1st – February 14th

PRESCRIPTION DRUG COVERAGE (Part D)

This coverage is available to all Medicare recipients. Stand-alone Medicare Drug Plans (PDP) supplement Original Medicare. The Affordable Care Act will be closing the "donut hole" that required seniors to pay more for their medications until benefits began to pay. It's predicted in 2014 that those that qualify will receive a 47.5 percent discount on certain brand name drugs and a 21 percent discount on generic drugs until they reach the out of pocket limit.

Medicare Advantage Plans with Prescription Drug Coverage (MA-PD) offer a variety of plans that members can choose from based on their personal health needs. Some Advantage Plans support and serve the prescription drug benefit, and some require their members to purchase from independent insurance companies.

Under the Affordable Care Act, 2014, higher income Medicare beneficiaries (those who earn more than $85,000 per person or $170,000 per couple) will pay slightly more for their prescription drug coverage. This change is expected to affect about 5 percent of beneficiaries.

These costs need to be included in any **Original Medicare or Medicare Advantage Plan** chosen.

LATE ENROLLMENT PENALTY

If you are new to Medicare and *DO NOT SIGN UP* when you are supposed to, you may receive an additional 10% increase in your premiums.

The Medicare.gov website actually specifies the following: "
    If you don't buy it when you're first eligible, your monthly premium may go up 10%. (You'll have to pay the higher premium for twice the number of years you could have had **Part A**, but didn't sign up.)

SHOULD I CHOOSE A MEDICARE ADVANTAGE PLAN?

Some seniors and families have found out the hard way that not all **Advantage Plans** are always "advantageous" for them. This decision can be very confusing to make, so let's make it as simple as possible.

The Insurance companies (the wealthiest industry in the world for a reason) are in the business of making and saving money. So they receive money from our government to provide services Medicare offers to their beneficiaries, at a profit. They also have extremely large marketing budgets, and sales tactics that can be very confusing to seniors and their families. First tip, the Insurance Company with the larger marketing budget is not necessarily going to be the Company that provides the most benefits.

Most states do offer a __DEPARTMENT OF ELDER AFFAIRS and possibly a SHINE program (Serving Health Insurance Needs of Elders).__ These programs are available to help guide and counsel seniors having to make this decision, and can be an excellent tool in counting the cost to determine which plan is the most "advantageous" route to take.

Some Medicare Advantage plans reimburse some or all of the Medicare Part B premiums, and many seniors struggling to survive on social security and/or shrinking pensions are often tempted to save money by joining one. Furthermore, if a beneficiary is in good health, they may receive many offers from different companies. The company benefits when their members are in good health, as they lose money by having to authorize costly hospital and specialty treatments.

In a nutshell ~ **MEDICARE ADVANTAGE PLANS ARE FOR HEALTHY PEOPLE.** So if you're in reasonably good health (no hospital stays, serious diseases, chronic diseases, etc.) they can be an affordable option, especially if there are no large assets or pensions to live on.

Seniors living strictly off of their social security income and/or social security disability income may qualify for their local state community Medicaid. One key change with the Affordable Care Act is that the local State Medicaid Program has been expanded, and many that may have been denied in the past, may now get approved.

Most State Medicaid programs pay what Original Medicare does not pay in co-payments, and prescription drug coverage. Many seniors meet the poverty requirements to be eligible for Medicaid in their state, however, have never applied.

APPLY, APPLY, & APPLY!

To be directed to your local state website:

www.medicaid.gov

(See Chapter 6 Understanding State Aid Programs)

CHOOSING A MEDICARE ADVANTAGE PLAN

First of all, if you decide to go with a Medicare Advantage Plan, you no longer have Original or Traditional Medicare, as that option has been waived. You may still have the red, white and blue card, so many think they still have Original or Traditional Medicare, but they do not.

What are the differences?

Members of a Medicare Advantage Plan are at the mercy of the Insurance Company they have chosen.

They will assign a **Primary Care Physician**, and most authorizations will go through that office. Any tests, procedures, specialist consultations, labs, hospitals, skilled nursing and home care will need to be authorized by them.

The primary care physician may have a "full risk contract" with the insurance company which means that the doctor receives a monthly amount per patient from the insurance company (usually $5 to $10 per patient), whether they see the patient or not. They can also bill for any patient appointments also.

In some cases, the doctor also receives more money if they don't authorize some costly tests, and/or Specialty consults. Some Medicare Companies also staff a nurse in the physician offices to issue authorizations to their providers for care.

Also, they usually have a **Nurse Manager** in the field that rounds on any of its members that are in any local hospitals and sometimes in their homes. This case manager will usually offer suggestions and decide what home care services or rehabilitation center therapies that a patient will receive.

So when weighing the cost of Original Medicare versus a Medicare Advantage Plan, weigh the costs very carefully. For a relatively healthy senior, this can be a good alternative to Medicare Part B premiums, however, understand that once there are hospital stays especially with any major illnesses, they will be looking for ways NOT to pay. This means there will be more out of pocket costs. On the first hospital stay or treatment for any serious medical condition, it's wise to disenroll from any Medicare Advantage Plan and return to Original Medicare.

The hidden costs to members that are in a Medicare Advantage Plan are usually discovered when a hospital stay, skilled nursing care, costly tests, therapy services or home care are needed.

For instance, a lot of seniors whom are in a Medicare Advantage Plan do not know that they will have a daily out of pocket co-payment at a Skilled Nursing and Rehab center, sometimes from day one, and will only be able to receive care at the Insurance Company's contracted centers (which may or may not be preferred).

If it's decided to go with a Medicare Advantage Plan, there are some quality companies. The locally owned companies tend to offer more consistent care benefits, however, may not be beneficial when traveling. Some local, not nationwide, Medicare Advantage Plans are owned by physicians, and may have the human compassion when authorizing needed medical services.

It's always best to get a wellness physical BEFORE you sign up with any Advantage plan to make sure that you know what, if any, medical conditions that will need to be managed by the company. It's for the patient's protection as well.

The large, nationwide Medicare Advantage Plans enjoy the largest marketing budget and the higher number of members, and have at times been the WORST at authorizing what their members require. How else could they afford the best marketing commercials, etc.? They make better profits when their members are healthy, not sickly.

When dealing with a Medicare Advantage Plan, you do get what you pay for. The more the company offers in the beginning, the less they will pay for later.

Also, the nationwide Medicare Advantage Plans usually have lower reimbursements for their physicians and ancillary providers, who are the trying to save money to maximize their reimbursement by not authorizing or providing the necessary services.

These are the doctors that routinely ask what Insurance a patient has when they see them at an appointment. A quality physician should be treating all patients according to the standard practice of medicine, regardless of their insurance.

Let me give you some examples, a 65 year old patient who had a hip fracture and surgery, found at the hospital that their Medicare Advantage Plan's primary care physician was refusing to authorize physical therapy in a rehab center due to the fact that the patient smoked, and wanted to send her home with Hospice, and throw in the towel. The family appealed, and won.

Another Medicare Advantage Plan's Nurse Case Manager refused to authorize skilled nursing care in a center on a patient who had a stroke because he also had dementia, which is a very common condition for seniors.

These are just a few examples of how they save money later, and under Original Medicare Skilled Nursing and home care therapies that are medically necessary are approved without need for any authorizations.

Usually under Original Medicare there are longer benefits that can be given, as long as the physician deems the patient requires it.

If a Medicare Advantage Plan is denying something that Original Medicare pays for, always appeal. If the primary care physician is in a "full risk contract" with the insurance company, they may be of little help. Legally they have to resolve an appeal within a specific number of days, given the circumstance, and the patient has the right to review their appeal decision. This process is not an easy one to win. That is why if it appears a senior will need intensive home care or rehabilitation services in the near future, Original Medicare is always the better option.

Many seniors think they will **NEVER** need any assistance in the future, near or far, and avoid any reminder of this fact. It might be human nature and a desire to live forever. The reality is that most illnesses are not a sudden surprise. There are usually gradual clues that a person is declining.

Any new medications prescribed for a serious medical disease is a sign of the possibility of needing more healthcare services in the future, and a good time to begin the disenrollment process from a Medicare Advantage Plan getting back on Original Medicare.

HOW DO I DISENROLL FROM A MEDICARE ADVANTAGE PLAN?

This can feel like quitting the post office, and can be very hard to accomplish.

The disenrollment period is from January 1ˢᵗ through February 14ᵗʰ annually. However, anyone is able to disenroll when they qualify for State Medicaid program, as well as if they're going into a skilled nursing and rehab center.

The customer service representatives are instructed to keep as many members as possible, and may not be very helpful. If possible, finding a kind hearted person in the doctor's office to help, as they usually have an inside person they deal with daily. Also, it's best to send multiple written requests to them by fax and certified mail. They will always process a disenrollment request easily once they think a member needs long term skilled nursing care, as they won't want to be having to authorize therapies, medications, etc.

Many people think that **Original Medicare** is too expensive, and may not realize that they are eligible for state Medicaid programs, depending on their monthly income, that may pay for Medicare Part B premiums, co-payments, and medications.

Original Medicare is still the easiest, open network with the most freedom to go to any physician, hospital, home care and Skilled Nursing and Rehab center.

Contrary to what may be said around election years, **NO PHYSICIAN IS GOING TO REFUSE A MEDICARE**

<u>PATIENT.</u> It's still one of the highest paying insurances in the country, with the least hoops to jump through. Only Concierge Physicians, which are generally private pay, will not accept Insurance Plans of any sort.

Original Medicare as a primary insurance, with a supplement (if it can be afforded) or State Medicaid as a secondary is the only and best way to be sure there will not be costly deductibles and co-payments due later.

Those inside the local healthcare community know that most physicians **WILL NEVER REFUSE A MEDICARE PATIENT**, regardless of whoever is the President of the United States!

In summary, count the cost carefully, and always try to get the most information from any Medicare Insurance professional that can help with the best prices.

For more information regarding Medicare Options:

800- MEDICARE   www.medicare.gov
                        Medicare Service Center

866-226-1819   www.cms.gov
Centers for Medicare & Medicaid

800-677-1116   www.eldercare.gov
National Agency on ELDERCARE

800-772-1213   www.ssa.gov
Social Security Administration

800-96-ELDER   Department of Elder Affairs

www.longtermcare.gov
US department of Health & Human Long Term Care

_____

*Fact: Many Seniors are not aware that Medicare will pay for
an Ambulance Trip to the Hospital.*

QUESTIONS TO ASK A MEDICARE INSURANCE AGENT

Can I continue with my primary care physician or will a primary care be assigned to me? _____ _____

What happens if I'm out of state and need healthcare?

_____

What hospitals, skilled nursing centers and home care agencies are contracted locally, and out of the area?

_____

Are there any daily co-payments if rehabilitation services are needed after a hospital stay? If so, how much and on what day do they begin? _____

Is there a "Tier Level" for authorizing Prescription drugs? _____

How much home care is usually authorized after a hospital stay? Is there only one company that is contracted, or will there be choices? _____

What is the disenrollment process, should I wish to return to Original Medicare? _____

What is the process to change a Primary Care Physician?

_____

CHAPTER 7

APPLYING FOR STATE MEDICAID &THE ROLE OF AN ELDER LAW ATTORNEY

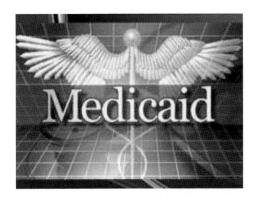

Medicaid is a "government insurance program for persons of all ages whose income and resources are insufficient to pay for health care."

(America's Health Insurance Plans (HIAA), pg. 232)

MEDICAID

"Enacted in 1965 through amendments to the Social Security Act, Medicaid is a health and long-term care coverage program that is jointly financed by states and the federal government. Each state establishes and administers its own Medicaid program and determines the type, amount, duration, and scope of services covered within broad federal guidelines. States must cover certain mandatory benefits and may choose to provide other optional benefits.

Federal law requires local states to cover certain mandatory eligible groups; such as qualified parents, children, pregnant women, older adults, disabled people with low income. States have the flexibility to cover other optional eligibility groups and set eligibility criteria within the federal standards. The Affordable Care Act of 2010 creates a new national Medicaid minimum eligibility level that covers most Americans with household income up to 133 percent of the federal poverty level. This new eligibility requirement is effective January 1, 2014, but states may choose to expand coverage before this date." www.medicaid.gov

Every state has a Medicaid program that was implemented in 1965 by President Johnson. Each year, national and local government leaders make changes to this program to include more or less services offered. Each state has an online and in person application process for these services that can include healthcare, food stamps, medications, mental health treatments, and case management for low income families and seniors.

A person doesn't have to be destitute to qualify for some or all of the services provided, and can be a big help, especially if a senior is living on a low social security disability / incomes. Some seniors have regarded state aid programs with disdain, viewing it as a handout. However, these services are what their taxes have been paying into, for many years.

Seniors struggling to survive on small monthly incomes and/or shrinking pensions can benefit greatly from these state programs. Most seniors have been paying taxes their whole life, and are able to reap the benefits of being a law abiding citizen and get the financial help when needed.

Under the Medicaid Program there are different categories for seniors eligible for Medicare. They are listed below.

<u>Medicare Savings Program (MSPs)</u> is for low income Medicare beneficiaries and is coordinated in conjunction with any state Medicaid benefits. Medicare beneficiaries may qualify for their local state Medicaid in a variety of ways based on their gross monthly income and assets.

<u>Qualified Medicare Beneficiaries (QMB)</u> will pay Medicare premiums, co-payments, and deductibles at 100% for those with a gross monthly income of $958, and individual assets of $7080.00 or less.

<u>Specified Low Income Medicare Beneficiary (SLMB)</u> will pay the Medicare part B premium for those with a gross monthly income of $1149, and individual assets of $7080.00 or less.

Qualifying Individuals 1 (QI-1) will pay the Medicare Part B premium for those with a gross monthly income of $1293.00 and individual assets of $7080.00, or less. This division is very dependent upon the availability of funding.

Low Income Subsidy (LIS) is available for prescription drugs and for those that are blind or disabled. These benefits can be accessed through the Social Security Administration office, or www.ssa.gov.

All of these programs can be accessed either online at www.medicaid.gov or www.benefitscheckup.org.

Every state has different local agencies that can assist with the application process, and they may come by various different names. In Florida, the Department of Children & Families assist in the Medicaid application process, however, many seniors have dismissed their help, reasoning that they no longer have children at home.

Regardless of the state, Medicaid is a program to assist those living at or under the federal poverty level.

Many states are implementing an initial online application, following with an appointment in person or over the phone. Any meetings in person with a state Medicaid office may require monthly bank statements proving any income and expenses.

Even if a senior receives too much in monthly income, and doesn't qualify for Medicaid, they may still qualify for food stamps or other services that can help ease the budget.

I met a widow struggling to make ends meet on a mere $800 a month social security, and had no idea how to pay for Medicare Part B premiums, and had not seen a physician in over 5 years. She had no idea that she qualified for her local state Medicaid. In her case, it was a decision of having to live with her family or remain independent in her apartment.

Each state has different requirements for the Medicaid program, however, many seniors that are struggling to survive, do qualify and have not known how to access these benefits.

Recently a family in Texas had their parents on a Medicare Advantage Plan, and their doctor would not authorize home care despite the desperate need for Dad, with an extreme care giving load falling on their mother. They both qualified for Medicaid, after disenrolling from the Medicare Advantage Plan they were on thus returning to Original Medicare, the same doctor happily arranged for the home care help they needed. Original Medicare with Medicaid as a supplement offers the most freedom for care options, with the least money out of pocket.

In another case, a senior had many frequent hospital and skilled nursing / rehabilitation center stays. The Medicare Advantage Plan had been reducing the amount of benefits they would offer her, yet she was suspicious of disenrolling from the plan. Ultimately, she agreed, and was eligible for full Medicaid benefits, received her therapy and was able to return home with full assistance under Original Medicare, and no money out of pocket due.

Getting past a senior's feeling that Medicaid is a handout can be difficult, but many have benefited by these state programs for years.

The very worst that can happen is that the application for Medicaid is denied.

APPLY, APPLY, and APPLY!

To be connected to your state's Medicaid website:

<u>www.medicaid.gov</u>

(Enter your State)

THE ROLE OF AN ELDER LAW ATTORNEY

Elder Law Attorneys offer a wealth of different assistance for families that want extra life care planning, especially if there are assets that will need to provide for a spouse for years to come.

They can assist with all estate planning, probate, tax questions, disability, long term care, legal documents, advance directives, healthcare surrogates, financial wills, trusts, Medicaid planning programs, case management, and guardianships.

Most elder law attorneys charge approximately $1,000 and more given the size of the income and assets involved. Many states do allow for personal need trust accounts to be established by family members so that a senior can qualify for Medicaid without depleting the family assets, especially if it may affect a spouse living in the community.

In some states, there are Medicaid Specialists that offer to help with setting up a trust and / or applying a loved one for Medicaid while preserving one's assets, especially if they are going long term into a Skilled Nursing Center.

If the income and assets are quite substantial, hiring an Elder Law Attorney is the wisest choice to protect those assets. They are experts at making sure all documents are current and accurate in accordance with the state laws.

Some families struggle when the assets have been depleted to under $100,000 and there may or may not be property involved. If an application to Nursing Home Medicaid may be coming, it's still wise to hire an Elder law attorney. Some have tried to hire a Medicaid Specialist in these cases and they've had to pay the state restitution and fines. Especially if there is property of some value, it's better to hire an attorney.

If a senior is going long term into a skilled nursing center, and has relatively low assets and no property, using a Medicaid Specialist can be a more cost effective alternative, as they have considerably lower rates than an attorney. However, choose carefully as many Medicaid Specialist companies are highly unregulated, and may not have the expertise they claim.

Be very careful researching Medicaid Specialists, as in most states, there's little or no licensure required, and many have claimed they could get the people approved on Medicaid, to no avail.

Board Certified Elder Law Attorneys are preferred, as they've received additional training and have a license to protect. Word of mouth, online research and checking with the State Law Board can ensure that you're getting a reputable attorney.

Elder Law Attorneys can also serve as a reliable partner to store a copy of Advanced Directives, Trust Accounts, and Financial Wills. They offer a neutral place that if any additional documents surface at a later date, the family can know which ones to trust.

You do not need to hire a lawyer to complete Advanced Directives, and usually any local Hospice organization as well as the websites listed below can assist you in getting these documents in place.

www.aarp.org/decide

To find an Elder Law Attorney in your area check below:

National Academy of Elder Law Attorneys
703-942-5711 or www.naela.org

CHAPTER 8

VETERAN BENEFITS for RETIRED MILITARY & SPOUSES

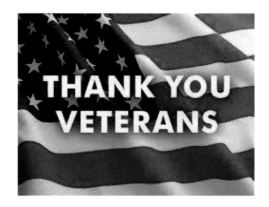

"As we express our Gratitude we must never forget that the highest Appreciation is not to utter words but to live by them."

John F. Kennedy

"It takes the courage and strength of a warrior to ask for help"

Author Unknown

VETERAN BENEFITS

Our veterans, regardless of age, many times are not aware of what benefits they are entitled to because of their service.

It has been astonishing to learn that for the men and women, who have sacrificed their life and safety for us, are not always aware that they have access to free to low cost co-payment healthcare at any local VA hospital, depending on their service connection status, and income criteria. Many get out of the military, and are never "debriefed" if you will, and some do not know benefits they are entitled to for life.

Some seniors have access to free or low cost healthcare at a local VA Hospital and never utilize it, either because they don't know they have this benefit or because they think they will receive substandard healthcare.

Most of the VA Hospitals are staffed with excellent medical professionals and are equipped with the latest medical tests, equipment and programs. However, some regions have better programs than others. Some VA hospitals offer a variety of specialty programs that are very unique and impressive.

Aside from having a primary care physician for care, veterans also receive free to low cost co-payments for any testing and medications they may need. They also can receive assistance for any mental health issues, such as Post Traumatic Stress Disorder (PTSD). For some veterans and their families, this is an extreme help to them financially.

The additional medical services veterans are eligible for are nursing, therapy, and social services in the home, oxygen, and medical equipment. The veteran has either free to low cost co-payments for these services depending on their service connection status and/or income criteria.

To get started at a local VA health care system it begins with enrollment. Veterans can now apply and submit their application for enrollment (VA Form 1010EZ) online at www.1010ez.med.va.gov/sec/vha/1010ez.

Veterans can also enroll by calling1-877-222-VETS (8387) Monday through Friday,   8 a.m. to 8 p.m. Eastern Time, or at any VA health care system or VA regional benefits office. Once enrolled, they can receive health at any VA health care facility nationwide.

Veterans will need their DD 214, and have been honorably discharged to receive access to the VA healthcare system.

Each VA system has a Care Management team (OEF/OIF/OND) to coordinate patient care activities and ensure that Veterans are receiving patient centered, specific access to care and benefits they're entitled to.

While many veterans may qualify for free healthcare services, most veterans need to submit an annual financial assessment, to determine if they qualify for free services. A veteran whose income exceeds the established limits, as well as those who choose NOT to submit a financial assessment, will have to pay required co- payments to be eligible for VA healthcare benefits. These co- payment costs per physician visit and medications are very nominal.

Certain services are not charged a co- payment at all. These apply to any publicly announced VA health fair or outpatient visits dedicated fore preventative screening such as vaccinations for influenza (flu) or specific diagnostic screenings, such as hypertension, hepatitis C, tobacco, alcohol, certain cancers, and HIV.

For some, a VA health care system may not be very close or easy to access. There is a reimbursement of travel costs that some veterans and/or their support system that they may be eligible for. In some cases, the VA will provide the needed transport (e.g. wheelchair van, ambulance when needed. Any transport eligibility can be coordinated through the Care Management team to determine if a veteran and/or their families are eligible for this service, and if any reimbursement travel costs are due.

Veterans and their families needing assistance to a wide range of information and services can also visit www.maketheconnection.net to find a place where stories can be exchanged, as well as information to connect to much needed assistance and veteran programs.

READJUSTMENT COUNSELING SERVICES

The VA offers readjustment counseling services through 300 community based Vet Centers nationwide. These counselors offer individual, group and family readjustment counseling to assist with the transition back to civilian life, however, also offer treatment for post-traumatic stress disorder (PTST), as well many psycho-social services including homelessness, medical referrals, employment, VA benefits, and the coordination of non-VA services.

Any Veteran that served during World War II, the Korean War, the Vietnam War (some territory exclusions), the Gulf War, and some of the occupations during a combat time period, are eligible for these services.

Vet Center Combat Call Center (1-877-WAR-VETS) is an around the clock confidential call center where combat Veterans and their families can talk about their experiences, and any challenges they're having in adjusting to civilian life.

MENTAL HEALTH CARE TREATMENTS

There are many programs that provide support for Veterans dealing with a variety of mental health illnesses. The programs range from primary care clinics, home based primary care services to general and specialty mental health outpatient and inpatient treatment health units.

There are specialty programs for those with intensive mental health diagnosis that include a specific case manager, social worker, nurse and psychiatrist. In addition, the veteran may be able to access rehabilitation and recovery centers, work programs and homelessness assistance.

We've seen a growing number of aging veterans that may be struggling without knowing they are entitled to these programs, as well as their support system to help manage behaviors and increase in health care needs at home.

Veterans that need access to trained mental health counselors can call the Veteran Crisis Lifeline 1-800-273-TALK (8255). This hotline is available 24 hours a day, seven days a week.

Those in crisis may text 83-8255 free of charge to receive confidential, personal and immediate support.

www.mentalhealth.va.gov VA Mental Health Benefits

AID AND ATTENDANCE PENSION BENEFIT

This program is one of the best kept secrets in America!

The Veterans Administration's Aid and attendance provides qualified veterans and their surviving spouse an additional income in ADDITION to any pensions they receive to pay for home care or assisted living care they may require.

The program is based on many different government criteria, such as the following: the veteran must have served active duty during a war, need assistance with at least one these daily activities: eating, bathing, dressing and hygiene.

They can be living either in a private home or an Assisted Living Facility, and need to provide written proof from a physician verifying the assistance needed, and meet the service connection level that is required.

This money is in **ADDITION** to the Veteran's service or disability pension, and any social security or disability money the veteran is receiving. The additional pay (up to $2,120 monthly) can be instrumental in affording the cost of medical care either in the home or at an assisted living center.

Each state has local **Veteran Benefits Officers** that assist at no charge in applying for this benefit at no charge.

There are also some companies that assist seniors and families in applying for this program at a fee. Any Elder Law Attorney would also be able to determine eligibility and help with the application process.

The veteran cannot receive this benefit if they require a **Skilled Nursing and Rehab center.**

Below is from the VA.gov website defining this program that senior veterans may qualify for.

"Aid and Attendance is a benefit paid in addition to monthly veteran pension and disability compensation. A&A can help cover the cost of in–home care, assisted living, or a nursing home.

This benefit may not be paid without eligibility to pension. A veteran may be eligible for A & A when:

- The veteran requires the aid of another person in order to perform personal functions required in everyday living, such as bathing, feeding, dressing, attending to the wants of nature, adjusting prosthetic devices, or

- protecting himself/herself from the hazards of his/her daily environment, **OR, The** veteran is bedridden, in that his/her disability or disabilities requires that he/she remain in bed apart from any prescribed course of convalescence or treatment, or, The veteran is a patient in a nursing home due to mental or physical incapacity,
- The veteran is blind, or so nearly blind as to have corrected visual acuity of 5/200 or less, in both eyes, and concentric contraction of the visual field to 5 degrees or less.

ELIGIBLE WAR TIME VETERANS:

- Served active duty during war time
- Are 65 years old, or older, or are disabled
- Meet the VA Asset Limit
- Have limited income and/or have extensive un reimbursed medical expenses
- Were honorably discharged
- A widowed spouse must have been married to the Veteran the time of the Veteran's death or have children by the Veteran and never remarried
- Physician order stating need for assistance

The program is available to any veteran who requires the "Aid and Attendance" of another person to avoid the hazards of daily life.

<u>Once Approved, Eligible Dependents Are:</u>

<u>The Veteran and one dependent</u>

<u>The Veteran's surviving spouse will be entitled to assistance in his/her retirement years.</u>

<u>2016 AID & ATTENDANCE BENEFITS*</u>

<u>Veteran Type</u>	<u>Monthly Maximum</u>
Surviving Spouse	$1,149
Healthy Vet/ Spouse Needs Care	$1,404
Single Veteran	$1,788
Married Veteran	$2,120

Aid and Attendance Benefits are currently tax free, and indexed annually for inflation.

*Please refer to <u>www.va.gov</u> for Annual Benefit Amounts (2016 Benefit Amounts Listed).

WAR TIME SERVICE INCLUDES

➤ World War II
December 7, 1941 – December 31, 1946

➤ Korean Conflict
June 27, 1950 – January 31, 1955

➤ Vietnam Era
August 5, 1964 (February 28, 1961 for veterans who served "in country" before August 5, 1964) and ending May 7, 1975

➤ Persian Gulf War
August 2, 1990 through a date to be set by law or Presidential Proclamation

LIST OF ITEMS NEEDED TO APPLY

- Military Discharge Papers – DD-214

- Married veterans and surviving spouses need   to provide a copy of the marriage certificate

- Surviving Spouses need to provide a copy of   the veteran's death certificate

- FORM: VA 21-2680 Examination for house bound status or permanent need for regular   Aid and Attendance

- Letter outlining monthly & annual fees paid to assisted living community or home care agency

- All Financial Statements

HOUSEBOUND BENEFITS

Like A&A, Housebound benefits may not be paid without eligibility to pension. A veteran may be eligible for Housebound benefits when:

- The veteran has a single permanent disability evaluated as 100-percent disabling AND, due to such disability, he/she is permanently and substantially confined to his/her immediate premises, OR,
- The veteran has a single permanent disability evaluated as 100-percent disabling AND, another disability, or disabilities, evaluated as 60 percent or more disabling.

A veteran cannot receive both Aid and Attendance and Housebound benefits at the same time.

Applying for Aid and Attendance and Housebound:

- You may apply for Aid and Attendance or Housebound benefits by writing to the VA regional office having jurisdiction of the claim. That would be the office where you filed a claim for pension benefits. If the regional office of jurisdiction is not known, you may file the request with any VA regional office.

- You should include copies of any evidence, preferably a report from an attending physician validating the need for Aid and Attendance or Housebound type care.
- The report should be in sufficient detail to determine whether there is disease or injury producing physical or mental impairment, loss of coordination, or conditions affecting the ability to dress and undress, to feed oneself, to attend to sanitary needs, and to keep oneself   clean and presentable.
- In addition, it is necessary to determine whether the claimant is confined to the home or immediate premises.
- Whether the claim is for Aid and Attendance or Housebound, the report should indicate how well the individual gets around, where the individual goes, and what he or she is able to do during a typical day."

www.military.com/benefits/veteran-benefits/aid-attendance-and-house-bound-benefits.html?comp=1199433946637&rank=26

VA HOSPITAL & MEDICARE

Even if a senior has full access to a local VA hospital, they may still need to be on Medicare part B for to cover physicians and procedures that may NOT be available at their local VA Medical System.

Many seniors qualify for community Medicaid, which can offset any medical expenses should they need them traveling or for any procedure the local VA Medical System cannot provide for the veteran.

The American Legion locally also host fund raisers for veterans that need assistance, or are struggling financially. The local legions can be a great resource to additional programs the veteran qualifies for, as well as an excellent place to save money on food and drink.

The chief reason to apply for benefits is because the government uses the total number of veterans approved for benefits as a baseline for allocating money for the health care programs. Even if a veteran decides NOT to use the local VA healthcare system, it can still reserve a spot for a veteran in need in the future.

Elder Law Attorneys can be helpful in applying for Veteran Benefits, especially if there are a lot of assets to protect, especially if a spouse that may need those assets for their retirement and care.

There are companies that try to charge for applying for Veteran Benefits, sometimes asking huge fees, however, this is illegal. There are local Veteran Service Officers that do NOT charge any fees to assist.

The only entity charging fees would be an attorney that is taking care of the entire estate, and they do not charge for the VA applications, as they know this to be illegal.

If an unlicensed person or company is trying to charge large consultation fees for this service, RUN! These people have no oversight, nor do they have a license or state bar to go to if they do not deliver what they promise.

FREE LOCAL VETERAN SERVICE OFFICERS CAN HELP LOW INCOME VETERANS APPLY FOR BENEFITS!

To Find a Local Veteran Service officer near you:

www.nacvso.org/find-a-service-officer

The links below can be utilized to see all veteran benefits:

http://benefits.va.gov/BENEFITS/factsheets.asp
Veteran Benefits Info

www.va.gov   VA Home Page

www.military.com   Military Branch Access
                                Website

www.nacvso.org/index.php   National Assoc. of County
                                Veteran Service Officers

www.vba.va.gov   Veterans Benefits Association

1-866-260-3274   www.caregiver.va.gov   Caregiver Support

855-260-3274   Veterans Affairs – National
                                Caregiver Support Line

800-273-TALK   Veterans Crisis Help Line

www.naela.com   National Academy of Elder
                                Law Attorneys (NAELA)

CHAPTER 9

UTILIZING LOCAL CHARITIES & NATIONAL HEALTH ORGANIZATIONS

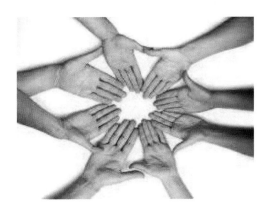

"The Universal brotherhood of man is our most precious possession."

Mark Twain

LOCAL CHARITIES

Every state and even every county within each state have different local civic and charity organizations. Some of these charity programs may be funded by the local governments, churches, or rely on local fund raisers.

These assistance programs may provide meals in the homes, nursing care, and transportation services to those that are homebound or are not able to drive.

Some of the states have had to make major cuts in their budgets and are cutting these charity programs that were extremely helpful in assisting those without health insurance.

Many disease based organizations that offer support group meetings will share information regarding local resources, free respite care, and even free medical screenings and services.

A lot of the local hospitals and senior centers advertise some of these programs when they are funded and available. However, some of these programs are only known to a select few working in hospitals. It's wise to attend some of the community educational lunches and programs that local hospitals offer for many reasons. For one thing, you may learn something new that will only benefit your overall health.

Secondly, establishing a personal relationship with a patient advocate or social worker that may have knowledge about resources can also prove beneficial for a variety of situations.

122

Knowledge is power, and the more that is known about choices and resources, the better.

The best way to find out about these local charity organizations is to search the internet with the key disease names or network with others locally. Also, social media can be very helpful as well.

Most hospitals have a facebook page, and if you "like" their page, you will be notified about upcoming seminars, screenings, and lunches. When you see an organization doing fund raisers at the mall, or other places, ask to be added to their email or mailing list.

If you or a loved one has a specific disease, make sure to register on their website and/or facebook page to be "in the know" on any upcoming events.

Some organizations provide meals, money, or free assistance to those that meet certain criteria financially or medically.

NATIONAL ORGANIZATIONS

The websites listed below are some of the national organizations that help people with certain diseases or conditions. For instance, some offer family members caregiver assistance; connect them with the local support groups and even money.

The Internet can be utilized to search any diagnosis that has been given, and receive information on local support groups and organizations that may have helpful programs.

When you or a loved one attends the support group meetings, you'll be in contact with people that have connections locally and nationally about all of the different programs these organizations offer. Since many of them receive federal funding, they can assist more people on a national level.

Years ago, the local Alzheimer's Association chapter provided free respite stays in an assisted living center for an Alzheimer patient, for a week or weekend. They would pay the centers directly. They also offered adult day care at no charge for families that needed a break from taking care of their loved one.

Once a person has been diagnosed with a serious disease, it's good to search out any national organizations that meet in the local area, and find out what resources they might be able to offer.

Below are some of the National Organizations that can offer support & education:

800-772-3900	www.alz.org Alzheimer's Association
800- 227-2345	www.cancer.org American Cancer Society
888.322.8209	www.epilepsyfoundation.org Epilepsy Foundation
800-223-27323	www.parkinsons.org Parkinson's Foundation
800-342-2383	www.diabetes.org American Diabetes Assoc.
202- 872-0888	www.n4a.org National Assoc. of Area Agency on Aging
800-222-2225	www.nia.nih.gov National Institute on Aging
800-677-1116	www.ncoa.org National Council on Aging

CHAPTER 10

ACCESSING MENTAL HEALTH RESOURCES

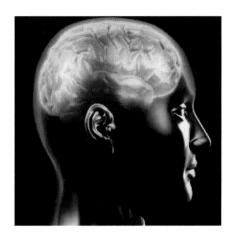

"Healthy Citizens are the Greatest Asset Any Country can have."

Winston Churchhill

FINDING MENTAL HEALTH RESOURCES

An estimated 26.2 % of Americans suffer from some type of mental illness, or 1 in five Americans 18 years old or older. Mental Health treatments are calculated at over 57 billion dollars annually in America.

The struggle families go through making healthcare decisions can be difficult in our system, however, it's even more difficult when there are mental illnesses and/or substance abuse involved.

For veterans there are a lot of support systems through the local VA medical centers which include nurses, social workers and physicians. There are comprehensive programs to assist with homelessness, counseling and medication management. The government also has transitional houses for veterans trying to get employment and get their life back on track.

Adults over 65 years old that suffer from mental illnesses such as depression, bipolar disorder, and schizophrenia, can have a more difficult time getting their healthcare needs met.

Thankfully, there is more awareness and preventative resources being offered than in the past. The Affordable Care Act has expanded resources available on a preventative basis for those managing any mental health condition.

If a loved one gets a diagnosis for any mental illness requiring medication, it's a good plan to file for disability with the Social Security Administration immediately, as they will eventually need that additional income and Medicare, especially since payment is retroactive to the first application date submitted. The earlier the application gets in the better.

There are many physicians that can direct a person to psychiatric counseling, home health and group homes. Some assisted living centers and skilled nursing centers cater specifically to those with mental illnesses and offer support groups and counseling on site.

With any mental illness diagnosis, the physicians need to be of the highest training and standards. Many of the newer trained physicians know the importance of counseling treatments along with medication management, not simply medicating their patients.

There are disability attorneys that can help with the application process, and usually will get paid when the benefits are approved, otherwise known as "on contingency".

Helpful website links may help:

http://www.ssa.gov/disabilityssi/ Social Security Disability Application Online

http://lawyers.findlaw.com/lawyer/practice/social-security-disability

OUTPATIENT RESOUCES

There are divisions locally through the National Alliance on Mental Health that offer support groups, education, case management and referral services for a wide range of age groups and disease types.

These programs also include assistance with substance abuse, which is increasing in our aged population in this country.

Most local agencies also have an outpatient case management program which includes weekly counseling from a licensed nurse or social worker.

Most of these services are offered at no or very low costs to the person receiving them. Some services are covered by Medicare, Medicaid or private health insurance.

To find out what programs are available simply go www.nami.org and put in a local zip code.

It's ideal when any mental health issues can be managed on an outpatient basis. However, this is not always easy to do without first having an Inpatient hospitalization.

INPATIENT HOSPITALIZATION

For some families it actually takes an inpatient hospitalization to identify fully the cause for any changes in behaviors, or mental health diagnosis.

An inpatient hospital stay can help identify and treat any underlying emotional or medical reasons why the patient is declining. Because some psychiatric hospitals offer separated age and sex units, it can give a senior suffering with depression or other illness the chance to see that they are not alone in managing their emotions.

Due to the improvement in psychiatric hospital programs and units, some agree voluntarily to go for treatment.

The other arrival scene for inpatient hospitalization is when a patient is "Baker Acted" otherwise known as a BA-52.

WHAT IS A BAKER ACT?

Under the Baker Act law, any law enforcement officer, physician, clinical psychologist, psychiatric nurse, or clinical social worker, can take someone against their will to a psychiatric facility for a mental health evaluation if the person is a danger to themselves or others.

A person can't be held involuntarily for longer than 72 hours, and a medical expert needs to examine the person and sign off on his or her release.

It's notable that the simple act of being held under the Baker Act doesn't mean the person is mentally ill or in need of commitment.

In 2010, less than 1 percent of about 140,000 involuntary examinations led to involuntary placement in a mental health treatment facility, according to the Florida Department of Children and Families. This number doesn't account for people who voluntarily remained in facilities.

Under the Baker Act, people who haven't committed crimes are not supposed to be treated as criminals and they do retain their constitutional rights.

In many cases the 72 hour evaluations by physicians and psychiatric professionals can help identify any medication management or other social service needs.

An inpatient hospital stay can also afford the family caregivers a respite, and identify if a change in environment is required.

CHANGES IN BEHAVIORS

A change in behavior can be a symbol of many things, both medically and emotionally. Simply because a senior may act differently does not necessarily mean they are suffering from a mental illness or any kind of dementia.

For many older adults, a change in behavior or dementia like symptoms can be a sign of a urinary tract infection, dehydration, or other medical condition that requires medical treatment at a hospital.

In a situation like that, after antibiotic treatment the person's mental faculties may return to their previous baseline.

Since depression in this country is increasing in our senior population, it's vital that a primary care physician be notified if and when there are any sudden changes in behavior or personal losses.

It's also important to have any **NEW** medications scrutinized and make sure that they are not creating a change in behavior, or any unpleasant side effects. Especially when there are multiple physicians treating an older adult, as one **Dr.** may be prescribing medications that are not cohesive to what they are already taking.

<u>It's crucially important at every physician visit that a complete and up to date medication list is included.</u>

Some families keep multiple medication listings so that if a senior is taken to the hospital suddenly, the medical professionals know exactly what they are taking.

CARING FOR AGING RELATIVES

The "sandwich generation" or those caring for their own families, while also caring for an aging relative are carrying a heavy load.

The guilt many adult children feel as a parent ages, needs more care, while denying that they do, can create confusing emotions. Some have confessed to having a "death wish" for an aging parent, and feeling guilty for having those feelings.

Many families struggle with the "when factor". When is the best time to talk with them about the care they need and who will take over financially.

Ideally it's best to work out these conditions early, before there is a need, and have a specific plan in place to honor the senior's wishes.

There are many caregiver relief organizations that can offer resources locally, as well as support groups to help a family member while caring for an aging relative.

Below are some of the websites that can offer information and local resources:

www.aagponline.org   American Association for Geriatric Psychiatry(AAGP)

www.alzheimers.org   Alzheimer's disease (ADER) Education & Referral Center

www.nami.org   National Alliance on Mental Health

www.nmha.org   Mental Health America

www.longtermcare.gov   US Department of Health & Human Service

www.mentalhealth.gov   HHS/Mental Health

www.samhsa.gov   Substance Abuse & Mental Health Services Administration

CHAPTER 11

PREVENTING SENIOR NEGLECT & EXPLOITATION

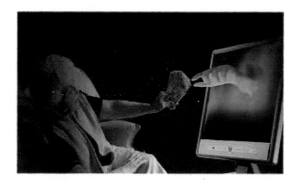

"Innocence is thought charming because it offers delightful possibilities for exploitation."

Mason Cooley, American Aphorist
1927 - 2002

WAYS TO PROTECT OLDER ADULTS FROM NEGLECT & EXPLOITATION

According to the National Center on Elder Abuse, Bureau of Justice, there were over 5 million reported cases of abuse in 2010. That means that 9.5% of the senior population reported some sort of neglect or abuse in that year. There is no way to know how many **UNREPORTED** cases occurred.

Of the reported cases of elder abuse 58.5% were for neglect, followed by 12.3% for financial exploitation.

Interestingly, 67.3% were females with the average age being 77.9 years old.

Fast facts:

➢ The average exploitation per reported case is $128,288.
➢ For those with mental illness, that amount climbs to $143,068. If Medicare costs are included, that amount climbs to $171,600.
➢ The closer the exploiter is to the senior, the greater the average amount will be exploited.
➢ The average loss per case when an adult child is the perpetrator is $157,326.
➢ The average loss per case when a family member is the exploiter is $125,193 (a 47 percent increase more than the average exploitation).
➢ The average loss per case when a grandchild is the perpetrator is $45,496.
➢ The average loss per case when a paid caregiver is the perpetrator is $18,350.
➢

➢ The average loss per case when the perpetrator has some sort of addiction issues (alcohol, gambling) was $25,688.
➢ The average loss per case when a stranger is the perpetrator is $30,219.

Methods of exploitation include both finances and property

Finances

➢ Scams
➢ Withdrawals from bank account(s)
➢ Cash
➢ Check (forgery)
➢ Credit Card (open debit card without knowledge, identity theft, or "borrowing credit or debit cards")
➢ Loans

PROPERTY

➢ Personal property
➢ House (stolen through transferring the property)
➢ Car theft or "borrowing"
➢ Rent (living off senior despite agreement)
➢ Medicaid (exploited senior now forced to be dependent on Medicaid

To prevent any financial exploitation, many banks offer seniors a third party oversight on any "shared" accounts, requiring the bank's approval on purchases. Many elder law attorneys also help in a third party role to oversee any real estate, or asset transfers.

Having a trained and trusted professional as a third party overseeing any financial decisions is the best way to guard against exploitation, regardless of how trusted a Durable Power of Attorney may be.

Too many seniors in our country are taken advantage of by people they know and trust. These can range from neighbors, church groups, television shopping shows, and most of the time, their own family members.

How does this happen? Sometimes, it's a gradual process.

Most seniors try to maintain their independence for as long as they can, many times much longer than is safe to do so. They may have family members or a support system that will NOT take advantage of them financially, yet many do.

Some seniors have a family member that has recently lost a job, or are going through financial difficulties and see caring for an aging relative as a meal ticket.

This section truly breaks my heart.

On a weekly and daily basis we would witness sons, daughters, neighbors that can't afford to live on their own, move in with an aging relative to "help them out", only to later take advantage of them financially. Many times a senior may need more care than the caregiver can offer, and may block help that is desperately needed.

Many state aid long term care programs, such as Medicaid in a Nursing Home or Assisted Living Facility, have a requirement that to qualify for the benefit, the state will pay all healthcare costs for the senior, however, any monthly income they receive must be turned over to the center.

When an adult child lives with an aging relative, some have forgotten how to live within their own financial means. The dependence on that senior's income and/or assets develops over many years and can become quite difficult to sever when the senior's medical needs change. When this transition has to happen, they may panic, and in MANY CASES insist they can take care of their aging relative although they are physically not able to.

This is usually evidenced by repeat trips to local hospitals, and physician visits.

Since most seniors insist that they will leave their home "feet first" if you will, relatives can tap into that desire, and actually jeopardize their health needs rather than lose the additional income they've now become used to living on.

Seniors with mental illnesses are especially at risk. Recently, a very confused and homeless senior was baker acted into a hospital, and then sent to a skilled nursing center for physical therapy. All she had as an emergency contact was a "friend" / former neighbor of hers. We promptly proceeded to set up a Professional Guardian for her, however, not before we caught him trying to apply for a credit card with her social security number. These situations happen every day, sadly.

For those that may be shaking their head, or thinking, that will never happen to me, or my loved one, consider this. Many have been affected by our uncertain economy, and in some cases, when an adult child loses their job, and may be in a desperate state, will insist they can take care of Mom or Dad, to get their monthly social security or pension, even if they are not able to meet their medical care needs.

One case, a daughter of a nursing home resident lost her job, and although her mother had been living in the nursing center for many years insisted that she could take care of her mother at home. The nursing staff that had been caring for her mother for years was alarmed, and her physician adamantly objected, however, the daughter insisted she could take care of Mom at home. I asked the daughter, "You do realize that if she dies, you will not be able to live off of her income any longer, right?" She, of course thought I was being dramatic. Her mother was dead within 4 weeks.

To witness a senior go through their final moments not receiving the care they need is horrific.

In one case the son of a 92 year old woman learned how to "work the system" efficiently. As the woman was declining at home with her son, he would bring Mom to a hospital, subsequently get some rehab for her at a nursing center under her Medicare (100 days) and still keep her monthly income. He would also get a break from caring for her. He would bring her home on the 101st day, and start the whole process over with a different hospital in another area. However, as her condition worsened, he became increasing desperate, and ultimately the state authorities had to get involved to remove his involvement in her care.

One remarkable 78 year old woman, who was very hard of hearing, had been living with her daughter for many years at the time. However, as Mom's care became more demanding, the daughter was getting more and more afraid, insisting that she not lose her mother's $1400 monthly income. She had developed a system though. She would put Mom in 2 diapers in the morning when she went to work, leave her some snacks to eat during the day, and when she returned home 8-10 hours later, put her in another 2 diapers to last her the night. Obviously she developed wounds and when the state authorities got involved, this very deaf woman wrote on a piece of paper "I don't want to live with my daughter!"

Many families don't live near their aging relatives, and as the senior needs more help in the home, may hire a person locally to assist. They may be recommended by someone they know and trust.

One such example was what an adult daughter referred to me as "Helga the Housekeeper." The daughter lived out the area and her mother hired "Helga the Housekeeper" for shopping and cleaning needs. She gradually began to get more involved in her mother's life. She went as far as to take her to the bank to add her name to Mom's bank accounts, and had been stealing family heirlooms that she claimed were "given to her". In this particular case, the bank notified the family of the attempted change, and financial exploitation was avoided.

HIRING A HOME CARE AGENCY

Many have made the mistake of hiring local help in the home only to find that the person has taken full advantage of their aging relative.

It costs more per hour to use a licensed private duty home care company, however, the staff they hire are usually bonded and insured, and had a positive background check.

Be very leery of private duty companies that have unfavorable state surveys, had many company name changes, and/or multiple state fines assessed. Since the more reputable companies do insist on a clean background check to work for them, the chance is better that their staff will be more professional, ethical and experienced.

There are opportunistic individuals that intrude into senior living communities and offer help to seniors, and especially if they think family is not living nearby.

Being proactive when an aging relative is needing help in the home will avoid them being prey to those that simply need a place to stay, or are in desperate need for money.

Statistics show that seniors living in Assisted Living centers live 3-5 years longer. This is due to the nutrition, socialization and nursing assistance. Therefore, when a caregiver for a senior is not open to this living alternative when they obviously require it, especially if it's being recommended by a physician, can also be a sign of some sort of possible financial exploitation.

This outlines the importance of trusting medical and financial decisions to the most responsible persons in a support system. They need to be financially independent themselves. Many seniors involve an attorney and / or bank officer as a third party to monitor both their finances and healthcare choices, just to be better protected.

The temptation by some individuals that have fallen on hard times to simply keep mom or dad at home when they are unable to take care of them, to have more income can appeal to those in a difficult spot financially.

Some cultures do not believe in a relative being taken care of by anyone except the family and I've personally witnessed families taking shifts to make sure their aging relative is taken good care of. These families are to be commended for their sacrifice, and great compassion.

Unfortunately, the opposite is what is being reported more and more. Since an elderly person can change so much as they reach their golden years, and can become much like a child, needing a tremendous amount of help, it's so important for families to have a **REALISTIC AGING PLAN**.

The families without a **REALISTIC AGING PLAN** are suddenly bounced around our healthcare maze, searching for answers and struggling to know where to go and what to do next. Hospitals have strict guidelines on how long someone can stay there, based on the insurance company involved, and will sometimes give families less than a day to decide on a rehab center, assisted living or home care support choices.

This is when the chaos and stress levels hit the highest levels.

What if you suspect that a senior is being neglected or exploited? Here are few signs that could mean they are vulnerable at this time or in some kind of a neglectful living situation.

➢ Frequent hospital stays
➢ Social Isolation
➢ Bereavement
➢ Become very suspicious
➢ Changes in ability to perform activities of daily living
➢ Has an overly protective caregiver
➢ Seems fearful or distressed
➢ Financially responsible for Adult Child or Spouse
➢ Depression or mental illness

Most states mandate that if you see or suspect neglect or abuse of the elderly to report it to the authorities at once. The take the alert anonymously, so the investigators make sure to protect the one reporting it.

If you suspect abuse of any human being, please contact **ADULT PROTECTIVE SERVICES   1-800-252-5400** (www.apsnetwork.org) or your local police department which can then connect you to the correct organization.

Below are some of the websites that offer additional ways to protect an elder from neglect and / or exploitation.

www.ncea.aoa.gov   National Center on
                                           Elder Abuse

www.aoa.gov 800-677-1117   Administration for
                                           Community Living

www.211.org   United Way

www.seniors.gov 800-333-4636   USA.gov

www.cmsa.org/800-216-2672   Case Mgmt. Society
                                           of America

www.caremanager.org   National Association of
                                           Professional Geriatric
                                           Mgrs.

www.caregiver.org 800-445-8106   Family Caregiver
                                           Alliance

www.longtermcare.gov   US Department of
                                           Health & Human
                                           Services

PROFESSIONAL GUARDIANS

A family suspicious of neglect or abuse for an aging relative, can also petition a judge to appoint a professional guardian. These are mediators that help protect those that need it, and have to report their findings to the court. They can also be useful to mediate a situation if differing family members can't decide on the right care for their relative.

Professional Guardians are sometimes called in when a senior has been the victim of neglect or exploitation. These are individuals that are ordered by a judge to care and make decisions for their "ward". Many times there has been family neglect or exploitation, or both, when they get assigned the case by the local authorities.

These individuals take a state mandated class to assist people that need some sort of assistance, either in healthcare choices or financial matters, or both. The difference is that all actions performed on behalf of one of their "wards" trusted in their care must be reported to a judge on a quarterly basis. They also are usually bonded and insured by the state, as most states do require this.

For some families that are disputing over the decision making of an aging parent (usually a wealthy aging parent) having a professional guardian involved can be a good alternative to family bickering. All parties would still receive an accounting of any funds used in the care of their relative and all involved can still visit and be involved however, there would be a neutral patient advocate, the Professional Guardian assigned, to make any final decisions that need to be made.

Most states and counties have an Elder Affairs department that can assist in contacting local Professional Guardians working in your area. Elder Law Attorneys work very closely with Professional Guardians and can be a great resource to find them.

www.guardianship.org National Guardianship Organization

www.naela.com   National Academy of Elder Law Attorneys (NAELA)

CHAPTER 12

HOSPICE, END OF LIFE, GRIEF COUNSELING & OTHER RESOURCES

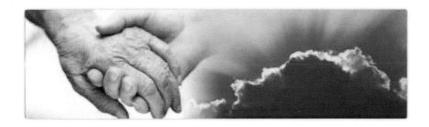

"You matter because you are you, and you matter to the end of your life."

Dame Cicely Saunders
Founder of Hospice Movement

In a very harsh and fragmented healthcare system, Hospice is the soft pillow for families to land.

Lengthy History of Hospice Care

Hospice: A Historical Perspective

The term "hospice" (from the same linguistic root as "hospitality") can be traced back to medieval times when it referred to a place of rest and shelter for weary or ill travelers, especially on a long journey.

The name was first applied to specialized care for dying patients by physician Dame Cicely Saunders, who began her work with the terminally ill in 1948 and eventually went on to create the first modern hospice, "St. Christopher's Hospice", in a residential suburb of London.

Saunders introduced the idea of specialized care for the dying to the United States during a 1963 visit with Yale University. Her lecture, given to medical students, nurses, social workers, and chaplains about the concept of holistic hospice care, included photos of terminally ill cancer patients and their families, showing the dramatic differences before and after specific care.

This lecture launched the following chain of events, which resulted in the development of hospice care as we know it today.

1965: Florence Wald, Dean of the Yale School of Nursing, invites Saunders to become a visiting faculty member of the school for the spring term.

1967: Dame Cicely Saunders creates St. Christopher's Hospice in the United Kingdom.

1968: Wald takes a sabbatical from Yale to work at St. Christopher's and learn all she can about hospice.

1969: A book based on more than 500 interviews with dying patients is published, entitled, *On Death and Dying*, which was written by Dr. Elisabeth Kubler-Ross. It identifies the five stages through which many terminally ill patients progress. The book becomes an internationally known best seller. Within it, Kubler-Ross makes a plea for home care as opposed to treatment in an institutional setting and argues that patients should have a choice and the ability to participate in the decisions that affect their destiny.

1972: Kubler-Ross testifies at the first national hearings on the subject of death with dignity, which are conducted by the U.S. Senate Special Committee on Aging. In her testimony, Kubler-Ross states, "We live in a very particular death-denying society. We isolate both the dying and the old, and it serves a purpose. They are reminders of our own mortality. We should not institutionalize people. We can give families more help with home care and visiting nurses, giving the families and the patients the spiritual, emotional, and financial help in order to facilitate the final care at home."

1974: Florence Wald, along with two pediatricians and a chaplain, founded Connecticut Hospice in Branford, Connecticut.

1974: The first hospice legislation is introduced by Senators Frank Church and Frank E. Moss to provide federal funds for hospice programs. The legislation is not enacted.

1978: A U.S. Department of Health, Education, and Welfare task force reports that "the hospice movement as a concept for the care of the terminally ill and their families is a viable concept and one which holds out a means of providing more humane care for Americans dying of terminal illness while possibly reducing costs. As such, it is the proper subject of federal support."

1979: The Health Care Financing Administration (HCFA) initiates demonstration programs at 26 hospices across the country to assess the cost effectiveness of hospice care and to help determine what a hospice is and what it should provide.

1980: The W.K. Kellogg Foundation awards a grant to the Joint Commission on Accreditation of Hospitals (JCAHO), to investigate the status of hospice and to develop standards for hospice accreditation.

1982: Congress includes a provision to create a Medicare hospice benefit in the Tax Equity and Fiscal Responsibility Act of 1982, with a 1986 sunset provision.

1984: JCAHO initiates hospice accreditation.

1986: The Medicare Hospice Benefit is made permanent by Congress and hospices are given a 10% increase in reimbursement rates. States are given the option of including hospice in their Medicaid programs. Hospice care is now available to terminally ill nursing home residents.

1989: The Government Accounting Office releases a study stating that only about 35% of eligible hospices are Medicare-certified. There are several reasons listed, one of which is the low payment rates HCFA had established for hospices.

1989: Congress gives hospices their first increase (20%) in reimbursement since 1986 and ties future increases to the annual increase in the hospital market basket through a provision contained in the Omnibus Budget Reconciliation Act of 1989.

1991: The Commission on the Future Structure of Veterans Health Care (Mission Commission) releases a report recommending inclusion of hospice care in the veteran's benefit package.

1992: Congress passes the Indian Health Care Improvement Act of 1992, calling for a hospice feasibility study.

1993: Hospice is included as a nationally guaranteed benefit under President Clinton's health care reform proposal. Hospice is now an accepted part of the health care continuum.

1994: HCFA sends a memorandum alerting the regions of problems regarding questionable certifications and re-certifications of terminal illnesses. This results in the first "focused medical review" for hospices and a wake-up call to the industry to improve its documentation and certification procedures or be denied payments.

1995: HCFA releases an expanded version of the Hospice Interpretive Guidelines, which provides much needed clarification of the Conditions of Participation (CoP). The Civilian Health and Medical Program of the Uniformed Services (CHAMPUS) Hospice Benefit are implemented June 1, 1995. It mirrors the Medicare Hospice Benefit in (CoPs) and reimbursement.

1995: The Office of Inspector General (OIG) announces the Operation Restore Trust (ORT), a special program to combat waste and abuse in Medicare and Medicaid in five targeted states—California, Florida, Illinois, New York, and Texas—would be expanded to include hospice.

1996: The Ninth U.S. Circuit Court of Appeals in San Francisco overrules a Washington State Law against physician-assisted suicide. The Second US Circuit Court of Appeals strikes down New York's law against physician-assisted suicide. Both rulings are appealed to the US Supreme Court.

1996: Bills are introduced in the U.S. House of Representatives and the U.S. Senate to make technical changes and improvements to the Medicare Hospice Benefit. The hospice industry provides full support for both bills.

1996: Major grant-makers pour money into funding for research, program initiatives, public forums, and conferences to transform the culture of dying and improve care at the end of life.

1997: ORT is extended and expanded to target all 50 states and additional types of health care providers.

1997: The Balanced Budget Act of 1997 (BBA 97) includes hospice provisions that, among other things, restructure the hospice benefit periods and remove physician services from the core services requirement. BBA 97 also reinstates a hospice cost report and reduces hospice payment updates by market basket minus one percentage point.

1997: Congress passes legislation barring taxpayer dollars from financing physician-assisted suicide. The US Supreme Court rules that mentally competent terminally ill people do not have a constitutional right to physician-assisted suicide, leaving the issue up to the states. Oregon voters affirm the right to physician-assisted suicide by passing for the second time its "Death with Dignity Act."

1997: The growing end-of-life movement focuses national attention on quality of life at the end of life as well as the need for increased public awareness and physician education. The hospice philosophy and concept of care are central to models for palliative and end-of-life care.

1998: Hospices nationwide report rapidly declining average and median lengths of stay. The percentage of hospice non-cancer admissions decreases dramatically, reflecting the problems associated with determining a six-month prognosis for these patients.

1998: An ORT report on hospice states, "Overall, the Medicare hospice program seems to be working as intended." The OIG reveals that hospice will not be included in the 1999 work plan.

1998: *Care Beyond Cure: Physician Education in End-of-Life Care* is released by the Annenberg Center for Health Sciences and the National Hospice Foundation.

1999: The U.S. Postal Service issues the Hospice Care commemorative stamp in February.

1999: The Health Care Financing Administration (HCFA) releases the Hospice Cost Report. Medicare-certified hospice programs must file cost data for each fiscal year on or after April 1, 1999.

1999: The Office of Inspector General (OIG) releases the Draft Compliance Program Guidelines for the Hospice Industry.

1999: The National Data Set Survey is initiated by NHPCO with the goal of creating standardized data collection nationwide.

2000: The National Hospice Foundation launches a four year public service campaign taking ads out to televisions and cable stations across the U.S.; one of these ads wins the prestigious ADDY Award.

2000: U.S. Senate holds two major hearings on end-of-life care that include discussions of barriers to access of hospice care under the Medicare hospice benefit.

2000: National hospice community calls for more consistent Medicare surveys

2000: The Duke Institute on Care at the End of Life is established.

2000: PBS series *On Our Own Terms: Moyers on Dying in America* is the focus of national education and engagement programs.

2000: Research from the Department of Health and Human Services, Office of the Assistant Secretary on Planning and Evaluation, shows statistically significant findings supporting the provision of hospice care for residents of skilled nursing facilities.

2001: The passage of the *Benefits Improvement and Protection Act of 2000* brings a five percent increase in the Medicare hospice reimbursement rates.

2001: A Call for Change: Recommendations to Improve the Care of Children Living with Life-Threatening Conditions is released by the Children's Project on Palliative/Hospice Services.

2001: The Health Care Financing Administration (HCFA) becomes the Centers for Medicare and Medicaid Services (CMS).

2002: The Department of Veterans Affairs launches program to increase veterans' access to hospice and palliative services while providing educational opportunities for clinicians in veterans' healthcare facilities.

2002: Rallying Points, an initiative of RWJF's Last Acts campaign, begins a three-year initiative to improve care and caring near the end of life.

2002: Federal court upholds Oregon's physician-assisted suicide law.

2003: National Hospice and Palliative Care Organization celebrates its 25th anniversary.

2003: A Clinical Guide to Supportive and Palliative Care for HIV/AIDS is released by the U.S. Health Services Resource Administration at The White House Conference on Palliative Care and the HIV/AIDS Global Pandemic.

2003: The web-based Family Evaluation of Hospice Care Survey is launched.

2003: The hospice awareness ribbon is unveiled prior to November's National Hospice Month.

2004: More than 1 million Americans with a life-limiting illness were served by the nation's hospices in 2004 the first time the million-person mark has been crossed.

2004: The Clinical Practice Guidelines for Quality Palliative Care is published in May by the National Consensus Project, a consortium of palliative care and hospice organizations.

2004: Elisabeth Kubler -Ross, a pioneer in the field of death and dying, dies at the age of 78.

2004: Robert Wood Johnson Foundation makes generous grant to National Hospice and Palliative Care Organization to advance public understanding and awareness of end-of-life care: NHPCO's Caring Connections is created.

2005: Caring Connections, NHPCO's consumer engagement initiative launches the comprehensive "It's About How You LIVE" national campaign.

2005: Robert Wood Johnson Foundation continues its support of NHPCO's Caring Connections consumer engagement initiative with an additional $4.9 million grant.

2005: The Department of Veterans Affairs releases the report, *VA Transforms End-of-Life Care for Veterans.*

2005: National dialog on the importance of advance care planning increases as the case involving Teri Schiavo, who dies in March, escalates in the media and within public policy debates. Having been a respiratory therapist herself, with no advance directives, her end of life became a legal family battle.

2005: The Diana, Princess of Wales Memorial Fund and the Franklin Mint make $3.35 million gift to promote better end of life care.

2005: The first national conference on access to hospice and palliative care is hosted by NHPCO in St. Louis.

2005: The American Heart Association and the American College of Cardiology release new guidelines about treating heart failure that includes recommendations that hospice care education be provided early in the course of an illness.

2006: Inaugural *World Day* is held on October 1 to focus global attention on hospice and palliative care; events are held in 70 countries.

2005: The number of hospice provider organizations throughout the country tops 4,000 for the first time.

2006: Quality Partners, a national, collaborative effort developed to build organizational excellence and improve hospice and palliative care delivery and outcomes is launched by **NHPCO** at the annual Management and Leadership Conference in New York City.

2006: The American Board of Medical Specialties (ABMS) recognizes hospice and palliative medicine as a medical specialty.

2006: U.S. hospice industry receives $13 Million Grant of Fujitsu Technology.

2006: A Guide to Supportive and Palliative Care for HIV/AIDS in Sub-Saharan Africa is released; the publication was funded by the U.S. Government through the HIV/AIDS Bureau, Health Resources and Services Administration, and NHPCO.

2006: Dame Cecily Saunders dies and a celebration of her life is held in Westminster Abbey on March 8; the U.S. hospice community issues a resolution honor Dame Cecily.

2007: Research published in *the Journal of Pain and Symptom Management* reports that hospice patients live an average 29 days longer than similar patient that did not have hospice care.

2007: Findings of a major study out of Duke University published in *the Journal of Pain and Symptom* Management shows that hospice services save money for Medicare and bring quality care to patients and families.

2007: The National Quality Forum releases *A National Framework for Palliative and Hospice Care Quality Measurement and Reporting.*

2007: The Alliance for Care at the End of Life, a 501(c) 4 organization is created to provide the hospice community with a more comprehensive, strategic voice on Capitol Hill.

2007: The Worldwide Palliative Care Alliance is formed to address global care needs at the end-of-life.

2008: The inaugural National Healthcare Decisions Day is held on April 16.

2008: The regulations (Conditions of Participation) for Medicare certified hospice providers issued by the Centers for Medicare and Medicaid Services were significantly revised for the first time since the original publication.

2008: Florence Wald, pioneer in the field of hospice care in the U.S., died peacefully at her home in Connecticut on Saturday, November 8. She was 91.

2008: NHPCO calls for increased access to palliative care in critical care settings.

2008: Certificate of Added Qualifications, or CAQ, in hospice and palliative care becomes available.

2008: NHPCO and its affiliate organizations (National Hospice Foundation, FHSSA, and The Alliance for Care at the End of Life) move into the National Center for Care at the End of Life in Alexandria, Virginia.

2009: The Accreditation Council for Graduate Medical Education, a private, non-profit organization responsible for the accreditation of post-MD medical training programs within the United States, adds hospice and palliative medicine to its list of accredited programs.

2009: The number of hospice volunteers continues to grow with a record 550,000 people serving as volunteers.

2009: *The NHPCO Standards of Practice for Pediatric Palliative Care and Hospice* along with the companion publication *Facts and Figures on Pediatric Palliative and Hospice Care in America* are released.

2009: Hospice leaders from the U.S. meet HRM Queen Elizabeth II at the Silver Jubilee Celebration for the U.K.-based Help the Hospices.

2009: Research published in the *Archives of Internal Medicine* suggests benefits of advance care planning discussions with physicians include lower costs and reduced utilization of aggressive care at the end of life.

2009: NHPCO's Caring Connections and Google Health partner to offer new way for people to access advance directives online.

2009: *Quality Guidelines for Hospice and End-of-Life Care in Correctional Settings* is published.

2010: *NHPCO Standards of Practice for Pediatric Palliative Care and Hospice* Receives American Academy of Pediatrics' Affirmation of Value.

2010: *We Honor Veterans*, a pioneering campaign to help improve the care Veterans receive from hospice and palliative care providers, is launched by **NHPCO** in collaboration with the **Department of Veterans Affairs**.

2010: A provision in The Patient Protection and Affordable Care Act will require state Medicaid programs to allow children with a life-limiting illness to receive both hospice care and curative treatment.

2010: Research published in *New England Journal of Medicine* finds that patients with non-small-cell lung cancer may live longer with hospice and palliative care.

2011: NHPCO publishes report, *Private Conversations and Public Discourse: The Importance of Consumer Engagement in End-of-Life Care.*

2011: *The Concurrent Care for Children: Implementation Toolkit* is released by **NHPCO** and the **District of Columbia Pediatric Palliative Care Collaboration**.

2011: Campaign for the National Center for Care at the End of Life Launched by National Hospice Foundation.

2011: Ethical Marketing Practices position statement and commentary is released by NHPCO.

2011: The bicameral Wyden-Roberts HELP Hospice Act is introduced in Congress. *The Concurrent Care for Children: Implementation Toolkit* is released by NHPCO and the DC Pediatric Palliative Care Collaboration.

2012: *LIVE—Without Pain*, a new public awareness campaign from NHPCO's Caring Connections, dispels myths about pain and empowers consumers.

2012: An innovative, online advocacy resource, the Legislative Action Center, is created online by the Hospice Action Network. More than 1.5 million people are reached through the six-part online video series, *Basics of Hospice.*

2013: Research from Mount Sinai's Icahn School of Medicine demonstrates cost savings of hospice and NHPCO and Hospice Action Network work to take this research to legislators and the media.

2014: Forty years after the creation of Connecticut Hospice, NHPCO and its affiliates celebrate 40 years of hospice care in the US.

2014: FHSSA expands its mission and is re-launched as Global Partners in Care.

*Prior article contributed from http://www.nhpco.org/history-hospice-care

WHAT IS HOSPICE CARE?

For many that have been diagnosed with a chronic and/or terminal illness, Hospice is a soft, kind partner for the journey. For those that are uninsured or underinsured they can be the lifeline of care that they would otherwise not receive. In short, Hospice in many cases fills in many gaps for those that need care in time of need. Since many Hospice programs are free or very low costing, they can be a beautiful resource for patients and caregivers in need.

Many people think that hospice care, or end of life care only applies to people that need **CPR**, or resuscitation.

In fact, **CPR** aka Cardio Pulmonary Resuscitation was designed for drowning victims. It's been historically very successful in saving an otherwise drowning patient that may be choking to death.

The truth is that **CPR** can be very damaging on an older patient with fragile bones, which is why the medical community uses it as a last resort, and only if a patient is dying, and is considered a 'Full Code".

Full Code patients have not put any advanced directive documents in writing, which means any and all resuscitation interventions need to be used. This can include cracking open the chest cavity to massage the heart, and other extreme tactics.

To put an older person through these harsh tactics can be avoided through education and many caregivers and older adults are seeing the value in putting wishes for their body in writing.

Hospice has programs that assist with end of life documents that are very specific and include pain relief measures that can greatly help any healthcare professional know how to proceed in an emergency.

These Advanced Directive Documents are crucial to ensure that a person can get or not get healthcare procedures as they wish.

The decisions they help patients and their caregivers face are a much needed help to any healthcare providers in their charge to know what and how to proceed in any change of medical condition.

HOSPICE BENEFITS

The main focus of hospice care is to allow an end of life patient receive comfortable care, and have an end of life experience that honors their wishes.

The programs have evolved from that initial goal to include community education, advanced directive document assistance, skilled and non- skilled home care, case management, medication management, much more.

The programs offered by local hospice companies depend on the funding and competition available.

In some areas of the country, hospice provides skilled home health therapies; physical, occupational, speech, IV therapy, and wound care. Usually these are paid for by Medicare, and there is no out of pocket cost to the patient.

Hospice benefits are very locally specific, and physician driven. When a physician gives an order to discharge a patient home with hospice benefits, the patient will be evaluated and receive what they are eligible, in accordance with what is offered in that area.

Most Hospice companies offer hospital beds, nursing home care, medication management, pain management, disease management, case management, comfort measures, respite care, palliative care, grief counseling, spiritual comfort, artificial feeding, nursing home and assisted living services and advance directive assistance.

They are leaders in community education on advance directives, and more importantly, having the discussions on a person's end of life wishes.

Although we still live in a "death denial" country, the importance of putting a person's wishes in writing cannot be understated.

When a loved one is in a hospital, has been given a chronic diagnosis, or had a sudden "unplanned event", the family and support system will have to make decisions on behalf of them. I've witnessed the agony they go through trying to make the best decision possible for them.

However, if they pass suddenly, and with no wishes in writing, they will second, third, and fourth guess every major medical decision made.

The seniors that put all these wishes in writing are giving their caregivers and family members the greatest gift imaginable, the knowledge of what they want, or **NOT WANT** to be done to them.

This becomes even more important in the event of a stroke, heart attack, or some medical event that leaves a patient speechless.

In this event, although the patient may have been admitted to a hospital for a urinary tract infection, pneumonia, or some other unrelated event, the end of life wishes in writing, aka advanced directives become the only way to be sure that the medical professionals are honoring their wishes.

Can a person change their mind?

Yes, it happens every day.

Some have filled out a **Do Not Resuscitate** form, however, coming close to death, have said "Save me", and if the patient is alert and oriented mentally, healthcare professionals will honor that wish.

Since none of us know **WHAT** decisions will need to be made at the end of our lives, it's crucially important all of us, regardless of our age and health conditions, make sure our advance directives are specific, and that we've also discussed our wishes with our healthcare proxy, or surrogate.

Hospice has evolved to include many other community based programs in many areas of the country. Some even include an HIV/AIDS program and counseling assistance programs.

Anyone who has been given a terminal and/or chronic disease should immediately contact Hospice to get enrolled in their system, even if there are no services needed immediately.

To find out what Hospice programs might be available to you in your area, check out the websites below:

To find a LOCAL Hospice Provider:

www.hospicedirectory.org   Hospice Directory Organization

www.nhpco.org   National Hospice & Palliative Care Org.

www.hospicefoundation.org   Hospice Foundation

To find a LOCAL Grief Counselor or Support Group:

www.griefshare.org   Grief Share

www.nationalallianceforgrievingchildren.org
National Alliance for Grieving Children

www.hospicefoundation.org/End-of-Life-Support-and-Resources/Grief-Support/Support-Groups

CHAPTER 13

HISTORY OF HEALTHCARE & THE LGBTQ PATIENT

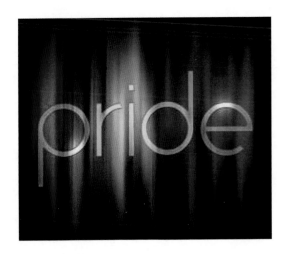

"If someone is gay and he searches for the Lord and has good will, who am I to Judge?"

Pope Francis

LGBTQ DEFINITIONS:

L – LESBIAN: Woman that prefers sexual intercourse with a Woman

G – GAY: General Term referring to a man or a woman that prefer sexual intercourse with their same sex.

B - BI-SEXUAL: Person that is open to sex with either a man or a woman.

T – TRANSGENDER: People whose gender, identity, or behavior differs from their birth sex or gender norms. (Female to Male FTM, Male to Female FTF, Cross Dressers)

Q – QUESTIONING: People who may be gay, straight or Bi-Sexual and still deciding or "Q" Questioning their preference.

LGBTQ can include people in any race, religion or financial status. It can be a relative, teacher, boss, fellow employee, authority figure or friend.

Why include chapters for the **LGBTQ** person in this book?

Because we are *ALL Aging in America*, regardless of our sexual preference, and they are our brothers and sisters, as one nation, under God.

The **LGBTQ** person will be referred to as "GAY" in these chapters, and Heterosexual person as "STRAIGHT", for simplicity sake.

DIFFERENCE BETWEEN SEX AND GENDER

Sex refers to the biological status of a male or female. These include the physicality of the sex, hormones, chromosomes, internal reproductive structures, and external genitalia.

Gender refers to a way that people act, interact or feel about themselves, which are associated with boys/men and girls/women.

WHAT ARE TRANSGENDER / TYPES?

In an overall description, Transgender is anyone whose identity, appearance, or behavior falls outside of the conventional gender norms. However, not everyone whose appearance or behavior is gender-atypical will identify themselves as a transgender person.

Transsexuals are transgender people who live or wish to live full time as members of the gender opposite their birth sex. Bruce Jenner is a common well known transsexual, considered MTF, or Male to Female. Biological females who wish to live and be recognized as men are called FTM, or Female to Male. They usually seek medical interventions, such as hormones and surgery to make their bodies as consisted as possible with their preferred gender.

Cross-Dressers wear the clothing of the other sex. Some cross-dressers do so to express their cross-gender feelings or identities; or for sexual arousal.

The vast majority of cross-dressers are biological males most of whom are sexually attracted to women.

Drag Queens and Drag Kings are respectively biological males and females who represent part-time as members of the other sex, sometimes to perform and entertain.

HEALTHCARE & THE LGBTQ PATIENT

The Lesbian, Gay, Bi - Sexual, Transgender, and Questioning patient population have experienced much discrimination in our healthcare system, and continue to in some states in America. Although there is much more social acceptance of people in this demographic of late, the healthcare community has lagged behind in the acceptance of these patient types.

Gay people have the same life experiences that the Straight person has; they work, own homes, look for and find loving partners, marry, adopt and raise children and also age in America.

They have many of the same problems anyone else does, with the exception that not all healthcare providers or the public have an open mind, spirit or adequate education in treating a patient that is Gay.

In some areas of the country, the employees may not be very warm and welcoming to a gay patient, and/or their partner and family, and in some extreme cases, have assumed that all MUST have HIV or AIDS.

Furthermore, because of the stigmas attached throughout the years, many gay patients are reluctant to discuss their sexual orientation with their physician or healthcare provider. The cultural and socioeconomic challenges many have faced for years also present hesitance in trusting their healthcare providers.

For instance, a straight woman can go to any hospital social worker or case manager and ask about the condition of their boyfriend/fiancé/husband and get all the updates they need to know.

I've personally witnessed a gay man or woman inquire of the social worker or case manager about the condition of their "PARTNER", and get what I refer to as the "Party Line."

The "Party Line" goes like this: "Who are you exactly? Do you have your Power of Attorney paperwork? I can't share any information with you as that would be a violation of the Health Insurance Portability and Accountability Act (HIPAA also known as the Privacy Act). I'm not going to risk my license without you giving us the proper paperwork."

The blatant double standard stemming from prejudice in the healthcare industry has been happening for many years.

This happens on such a frequent basis that many cities in our county are registering gay couples and issuing the paperwork that "some" healthcare professionals need to disclose information to in the event of a medical emergency.

Since our nation is becoming more accepting of people and their sexual preferences, older gay couples are feeling comfortable to come out publicly about their relationships and get married, if their state allows. Since so many states are legalizing gay marriage, and finally allowing them to have the same privilege that straight married couples enjoy, there is more need for gay couples to know how to protect themselves legally, financially, and medically.

These chapters are for the LGBTQ / Gay community; regardless of their age navigate our healthcare system as they age in America.

It's also meant to help the healthcare community and others understand the history they've endured, and hopefully inspire understanding and compassion.

Quote from Pope Francis "If someone is gay and searches for the Lord and has goodwill, who am I to judge?"

Taking the lead of Pope Francis, we could all ask ourselves "Who am I to judge?"

<u>HISTORY OF GAY RIGHTS</u>

The American Gay Rights Movement: A Timeline*

*This timeline provides information about the gay rights movement in the United States from 1924 to the present: including the Stonewall riots; the contributions of Harvey Milk; the "Don't Ask, Don't Tell" policy; the first civil unions; the legalization of same-sex marriage in Massachusetts, Connecticut, New York; and more.

1924

The Society for Human Rights in Chicago becomes the country's earliest known gay rights organization.

1948

<u>Alfred Kinsey</u> publishes *Sexual Behavior in the Human Male*, revealing to the public that homosexuality is far more widespread than was commonly believed.

1951

The Mattachine Society, the first national gay rights organization, is formed by Harry Hay, considered by many to be the founder of the gay rights movement.

1955

The first lesbian-rights organization in the United States, the Daughters of Bilitis, was established in San Francisco in 1955.

1956

The Daughters of Bilitis, a pioneering national lesbian organization, is founded.

1958

Joe Cino, an Italian-American theater producer, opens Caffe Cino. Caffe Cino is credited with starting the Off-Off-Broadway theater movement. Six years after Caffe Cino opens, it hosts the first gay plays, *The Madness of Lady Bright*, by <u>Lanford Wilson</u>, and *The Haunted Host*, by Robert Patrick.

1962

Illinois becomes the first state in the U.S. to decriminalize homosexual acts between consenting adults in private.

1966

The world's first the transgender organization, the National Transsexual Counseling Unit, was established in San Francisco.

1969

The Stonewall riots transform the gay rights movement from one limited to a small number of activists into a widespread protest for equal rights and acceptance. Patrons of a gay bar in New York's Greenwich Village, the Stonewall Inn, fight back during a police raid on **June 27**, sparking three days of riots.

1973

The American Psychiatric Association removes homosexuality from its official list of mental disorders.

<u>Harvey Milk</u> runs for city supervisor in San Francisco. He runs on a socially liberal platform and opposes government involvement in personal sexual matters. Milk comes in 10th out of 32 candidates, earning 16,900 votes, winning the Castro District and other liberal neighborhoods. He receives a lot of media attention for his passionate speeches, brave political stance, and media skills.

1976

San Francisco Mayor George Moscone appoints Harvey Milk to the Board of Permit Appeals, making Milk the first openly gay city commissioner in the United States. Milk decides to run for the California State Assembly and Moscone is forced to fire him from the Board of Permit Appeals after just five weeks. Milk loses the State Assembly race by fewer than 4,000 votes. Believing the Alice B. Toklas LGBT Democratic Club will never support him politically, Milk co-founds the San Francisco Gay Democratic Club after his election loss.

1977

Activists in Miami, Florida pass a civil rights ordinance making sexual orientation discrimination illegal in Dade County. *Save Our Children*, a campaign by a Christian fundamentalist group and headed by singer Anita Bryant, is launched in response to the ordinance. In the largest special election of any in Dade County history, 70% vote to overturn the ordinance. It is a crushing defeat for gay activists.

1978

On **January 8**, Harvey Milk makes national news when he is sworn in as a member of the San Francisco Board of Supervisors. Running against 16 other candidates, he wins the election by 30 percent. Milk begins his term by sponsoring a civil rights bill that outlaws sexual orientation discrimination. Only one supervisor votes against it and Mayor Moscone signs it into law.

John Briggs drops out of the California governor's race, but receives support for Proposition 6, also known as the Briggs Initiative, a proposal to fire any teacher or school employee who publicly supports gay rights. Harvey Milk campaigns against the bill and attends every event hosted by Briggs. In the summer, attendance greatly increases at Gay Pride marches in San Francisco and Los Angeles, partly in response to Briggs. President Jimmy Carter,

Former Governor Ronald Reagan and Governor Jerry Brown speak out against the proposition. On **November 7**, voters reject the proposition by more than a million votes.

On **November 27**, Harvey Milk and Mayor George Moscone are assassinated by Dan White, another San Francisco city supervisor, who had recently resigned and wanted his job back, but was being passed over because he wasn't the best fit for the liberal leaning Board of Supervisors and the ethnic diversity in White's district. San Francisco pays tribute to Harvey Milk by naming several locations after him, included Harvey Milk Plaza at the intersection of Market and Castro streets. The San Francisco Gay Democratic Club changes its name to the Harvey Milk Memorial Gay Democratic Club.

1979

About 75,000 people participated in the National March on Washington for Lesbian and Gay Rights in Washington, D.C., in October. It was the largest political gathering in support of LGBT rights to date.

1980

At the 1980 Democratic National Convention held at New York City's Madison Square Garden, Democrats took a stance supporting gay rights, adding the following to their plank: "All groups must be protected from discrimination based on race, color, religion, national origin, language, age, sex or sexual orientation."

1982

Wisconsin becomes the first state to outlaw discrimination on the basis of sexual orientation.

1984

The city of Berkeley, California, becomes the first city to offer its employees domestic-partnership benefits.

1993

The "Don't Ask, Don't Tell" policy is instituted for the U.S. military, permitting gays to serve in the military but banning homosexual activity. President Clinton's original intention to revoke the prohibition against gays in the military was met with stiff opposition; this compromise, which has led to the discharge of thousands of men and women in the armed forces, was the result. On **April 25**, an estimated 800,000 to one million people participate in the March on Washington for Lesbian, Gay, and Bi Equal Rights and Liberation. Several events such as art and history exhibits, public service outings and workshops are held throughout Washington, DC leading up the event. Jesse Jackson, RuPaul, Martina Navratilova, and Eartha Kitt are among the speakers and performers at a rally after the march. The march is a response to "Don't Ask Don't Tell", Amendment 2 in Colorado, as well as rising hate crimes and ongoing discrimination against the LGBT community.

1996

In *Romer* v. *Evans*, the Supreme Court strikes down Colorado's Amendment 2, preventing protected status based upon homosexuality or bisexuality did not satisfy the Equal Protection Clause. According to Justice Anthony Kennedy, "We find nothing special in the protections Amendment 2 withholds. These protections . . . constitute ordinary civil life in a free society."

2000

Vermont becomes the first state in the country to legally recognize civil unions between gay or lesbian couples. The law states that these "couples would be entitled to the same benefits, privileges, and responsibilities as spouses." It stops short of referring to same-sex unions as marriage, which the state defines as heterosexual.

2003

The U.S. Supreme Court rules in _Lawrence_ v. _Texas_ that sodomy laws in the U.S. are unconstitutional. Justice Anthony Kennedy wrote, "Liberty presumes an autonomy of self that includes freedom of thought, belief, expression, and certain intimate conduct."

In **November**, the Massachusetts Supreme Judicial Court ruled that barring gays and lesbians from marrying violates the state constitution. The Massachusetts Chief Justice concluded that to "deny the protections, benefits, and obligations conferred by civil marriage" to gay couples was unconstitutional because it denied "the dignity and equality of all individuals" and made them "second-class citizens." Strong opposition followed the ruling.

2004

On **May 17**, same-sex marriages become legal in Massachusetts.

2005

Civil unions become legal in Connecticut in **October**.

2006

Civil unions become legal in New Jersey in **December**.

2007

In **November**, the House of Representatives approves a bill ensuring equal rights in the workplace for gay men, lesbians, and bisexuals.

2008

In **February**, a New York State appeals court unanimously votes that valid same-sex marriages performed in other states must be recognized by employers in New York, granting same-sex couples the same rights as other couples.

In **February**, the state of Oregon passes a law that allows same-sex couples to register as domestic partners allowing them some spousal rights of married couples.

180

On **May 15**, the California Supreme Court rules that same-sex couples have a constitutional right to marry. By

November 3rd, more than 18,000 same-sex couples have married. On November 4, California voters approved a ban on same-sex marriage called Proposition 8. The attorney general of California, Jerry Brown, asked the state's Supreme Court to review the constitutionality of Proposition 8. The ban throws into question the validity of the more than 18,000 marriages already performed, but

Attorney General Brown reiterated in a news release that he believed the same-sex marriages performed in California before November 4 should remain valid, and the California Supreme Court, which upheld the ban in May 2009, agreed, allowing those couples married under the old law to remain that way.
November 4, voters in California, Arizona, and Florida approved the passage of measures that ban same-sex marriage. Arkansas passed a measure intended to bar gay men and lesbians from adopting children.
On **October 10**, the Supreme Court of Connecticut rules that same-sex couples have the right to marry. This makes Connecticut the second state, after Massachusetts, to legalize civil marriage for same-sex couples. The court rules that the state cannot deny gay and lesbian couples the freedom to marry under Connecticut's constitution, and that the state's civil union law does not provide same-sex couples with the same rights as heterosexual couples.
On **November 12**, same-sex marriages begin to be officially performed in Connecticut.

2009

On **April 3**, the Iowa Supreme Court unanimously rejects the state law banning same-sex marriage. Twenty-one days later, county recorders are required to issue marriage licenses to same-sex couples.
On **April 7**, the Vermont Legislature votes to override Gov. Jim Douglas's veto of a bill allowing gays and lesbians to marry, legalizing same-sex marriage. It is the first state to

legalize gay marriage through the legislature; the courts of the other states in which the marriage is legal—Massachusetts, Connecticut, and Iowa—gave approval.

On **May 6**, the governor of Maine legalized same-sex marriage in that state in Maine; however, citizens voted to overturn that law when they went to the polls in November, and Maine became the 31st state to ban the practice.

On **June 3**, New Hampshire governor John Lynch signs legislation allowing same-sex marriage. The law stipulates that religious organizations and their employees will not be required to participate in the ceremonies. New Hampshire is the sixth state in the nation to allow same-sex marriage.

On **June 17**, President Obama signs a referendum allowing the same-sex partners of federal employees to receive benefits. They will not be allowed full health coverage, however. This is Obama's first major initiative in his campaign promise to improve gay rights.

On **August 12**, President Obama posthumously awards Harvey Milk the Presidential Medal of Freedom.

2010

March 3, Congress approves a law signed in December 2009 that legalizes same-sex marriage in the District of Columbia.

August 4, Chief U.S. District Judge Vaughn Walker rules that Proposition 8, the 2008 referendum that banned same-sex marriage in California, violates the 14th Amendment's equal protection clause. "Proposition 8 singles out gays and lesbians and legitimates their unequal treatment," Vaughn writes. "Proposition 8 perpetuates the stereotype that gays and lesbians are incapable of forming long-term loving relationships and that gays and lesbians are not good parents."

December 18, the U.S. Senate votes 65 to 31 in favor of repealing Don't Ask, Don't Tell, the Clinton-era military policy that forbids openly gay men and women from serving in the military. Eight Republicans side with the Democrats to strike down the ban. The ban will not be lifted officially until President Obama, Defense Secretary Robert Gates, and Admiral Mike Mullen, the chairman of the Joint Chiefs of Staff, agree that the military is ready to enact the change and that it won't affect military readiness. On **Dec. 18**,

President Obama officially repeals the "Don't Ask, Don't Tell" military policy.

2011

June 24, New York passes a law to allow same-sex marriage. New York is now the largest state that allows gay and lesbian couples to marry. The vote comes on the eve of the city's annual Gay Pride Parade and gives new momentum to the national gay-rights movement. The marriage bill is approved with a 33 to 29 vote. Cheering supporters greet Gov. Andrew Cuomo as he arrives on the Senate floor to sign the measure at 11:55pm, just moments after the vote. After making same-sex marriage one of his top priorities, Cuomo emerges as a true champion of gay rights.

2012

February 7, the Ninth Circuit Court of Appeals in California rules 2–1 that Proposition 8, the 2008 referendum that banned same-sex marriage in state, is unconstitutional because it violates the Equal Protection Clause of the 14th Amendment. In the ruling, the court says, the law "operates with no apparent purpose but to impose on gays and lesbians, through the public law, a majority's private disapproval of them and their relationships."

February 13, Washington becomes the seventh state to legalize gay marriage.

March 1, Maryland passes legislation to legalize gay marriage, becoming the eighth state to do so.

May 9, President Barack Obama endorses same-sex marriage. "It is important for me to go ahead and affirm that I think same-sex couples should be able to get married," he said. He makes the statement days after Vice President Joe Biden and Secretary of Education Arne Duncan both came out in support of gay marriage.

Nov. 6, Tammy Baldwin, a seven-term Democratic congresswoman from Wisconsin, prevails over former governor Tommy Thompson in the race for U.S. Senate and becomes the first openly gay politician elected to the Senate. Also on Election Day, gay marriage is approved in a popular vote for the first time. Maine and Maryland vote in favor of allowing same-sex marriage.

In addition, voters in Minnesota reject a measure to ban same-sex marriage.

2013

Feb. 27, in a policy shift for party members, several Republicans back a legal brief asking the Supreme Court to rule that same-sex marriage is a constitutional right. More than 100 Republicans are listed on the brief, including former New Hampshire Congressman Charles Bass and Beth Myers. Myers was a key adviser to Mitt Romney during his 2012 presidential campaign. The brief is filed as the U.S. Supreme Court prepares to consider overturning Proposition 8, the California initiative banning same-sex marriage, as well as overturning the Defense of Marriage Act, a federal law passed during Bill Clinton's presidency, which defines marriage as between a man and a woman.

March 26, the Supreme Court begins two days of historical debate over gay marriage. During the debate, the Supreme Court consider overturning Proposition 8, the California initiative banning same-sex marriage, and the Defense of Marriage Act, a federal law passed during Bill Clinton's presidency, which defines marriage as between a man and a woman. The Supreme Court's decision will be announced in June 2013.

April 29, Jason Collins of the NBA's Washington Wizards announces in an essay in *Sports Illustrated* that he is gay. "I'm a 34-year-old N.B.A. center. I'm black and I'm gay," he writes. "I've reached that enviable state in life in which I can do pretty much what I want. And what I want is to continue to play basketball. I still love the game, and I still have something to offer. My coaches and teammates recognize that. At the same time, I want to be genuine and authentic and truthful." Collins is the first active athlete in the NBA, NFL, NHL, or MLB to make the announcement.

May 2, after same-sex marriage legislation passes in both houses of Rhode Island's legislature, Governor Lincoln Chafee signs it into law. The new law, legalizing same-sex marriage, goes into effect on August 1, 2013.

May 7, Governor Jack Markell signs the Civil Marriage Equality and Religious Freedom act, legalizing same-sex marriage for the state of Delaware. The new law goes into effect on July 1, 2013.

May 13, in Minnesota, the State Senate votes 37 to 30 in favor of legalizing same-sex marriage. The vote comes a week after it passes in the House. Governor Mark Dayton, a supporter of same-sex marriage, says he will sign the bill the following afternoon. Gay couples will be able to marry in Minnesota in August 2013.

June 26, the Supreme Court rules that the 1996 Defense of Marriage Act (DOMA) is unconstitutional. In a 5 to 4 vote, the court rules that DOMA violates the rights of gays and lesbians. The court also rules that the law interferes with the states' rights to define marriage. It is the first case ever on the issue of gay marriage for the Supreme Court. Chief Justice John G. Roberts, Jr. votes against striking it down as does Antonin Scalia, Samuel Alito and Clarence Thomas. However, conservative-leaning Justice Anthony M. Kennedy votes with his liberal colleagues to overturn DOMA.

July 17, Queen Elizabeth II approves a same-sex marriage bill for England and Wales. Her approval comes a day after it passes in Parliament. While the queen's approval is simply a formality, her quick response clears the way for the first gay marriages to happen as soon as 2014 in England and Wales. The bill allows same-sex couples to marry in both religious and civil ceremonies. It also allows couples currently in a civil partnership to convert it into a marriage. Scotland is currently considering its own new legislation on same-sex marriage.

Aug. 1, Minnesota and Rhode Island begin issuing marriage licenses to same-sex couples this month.

Oct. 21, in a unanimous vote, the New Jersey Supreme Court rejects Gov. Chris Christie's request to delay the implementation date of same-sex weddings. Same-sex couples in New Jersey begin to marry. Just hours later, Christie drops his appeal to legalize same-sex marriages. Therefore, New Jersey becomes the 14th state to recognize same-sex marriages.

Nov. 5, Illinois becomes the 15th state to recognize same-sex marriages when the House of Representatives approve the Religious Freedom and Marriage Fairness Act, which passed the state Senate in February 2013. Governor Pat Quinn, a strong supporter of same-sex marriage, will sign it into law. The new law will be implemented on June 1, 2014.

Nov. 12, Hawaii becomes the 16th state to recognize same-sex marriages when the Senate passes a gay marriage bill, which had already passed in the House. Governor Neil Abercrombie, a vocal supporter of gay marriage, says he will sign the bill. Beginning December 2, gay couples who are residents of Hawaii as well as tourists can marry in the state. Hawaii is already a very popular state for destination weddings. State Senator J. Kalani English says, "This is nothing more than the expansion of aloha in Hawaii." To see a current list of all the states that have legalized same-sex marriage, go here.

2014

Jan. 6, The United States Supreme Court blocks any further same-sex marriages in Utah while state officials appeal the decision made by Judge Shelby in late December 2013. The block creates legal limbo for the 1,300 same-sex couples who have received marriage licenses since Judge Shelby's ruling.

Jan. 10, The Obama administration announces that the federal government will recognize the marriages of the 1,300 same-sex couples in Utah even though the state government has currently decided not to do so. In a video announcement on the Justice Department website, Attorney General Eric Holder says, "I am confirming today that, for purposes of federal law, these marriages will be recognized as lawful and considered eligible for all relevant federal benefits on the same terms as other same-sex marriages. These families should not be asked to endure uncertainty regarding their status as the litigation unfolds." With federal approval, same-sex couples will be able to receive spousal benefits, like health insurance for federal employees and filing joint federal income tax returns.

May 19, Same-sex marriage becomes legal in Oregon when a U.S. federal district judge rules that the state's 2004 constitutional amendment banning same-sex marriage violates the Equal Protection clause in the U.S. Constitution.

May 20, A judge strikes down the same-sex marriage ban in Pennsylvania, making the state the 18th to legalize gay marriage. The judge rules that Pennsylvania's 1996 ban on same-sex marriage is unconstitutional. The state is the last in the Northeast to legalize same-sex marriage. Before now, the state did not even recognize domestic partnerships or civil unions.

Oct. 6, The U.S. Supreme Court declines to hear appeals of rulings in Indiana, Oklahoma, Utah, Virginia, and Wisconsin that allowed same-sex marriage. The move paves the way for same-sex marriages in the five states. In fact, Virginia announced that unions would begin that day.

Nov. 12, The U.S. Supreme Court denies a request to block same-sex marriage in Kansas.

Nov. 19, A federal judge strikes down Montana's ban that same-sex marriage is unconstitutional.

Nov. 20, The U.S. Supreme Court denies a request to block same-sex marriage in South Carolina. The ruling means South Carolina becomes the 35th U.S. state where same-sex marriage is legal.

2015

June 26, The U.S. Supreme Court ruled, 5–4, in *Obergefell v. Hodges* that same-sex couples have the fundamental right to marry and that states cannot say that marriage is reserved for heterosexual couples. "Under the Constitution, same-sex couples seek in marriage the same legal treatment as opposite-sex couples, and it would disparage their choices and diminish their personhood to deny them this right," Justice Anthony Kennedy wrote in the majority opinion.

July 27, The Boy Scouts of America (BSA) ended its ban on gay adult leaders. The new policy was approved by the BSA National Executive Board by a 45-12 vote. The new policy did still allow church-sponsored Scout groups to ban gay adults for religious reasons.

*Article excerpted from
http://www.infoplease.com/ipa/A0761909.html

In a landmark ruling issued in June, the U.S. Supreme Court ruled that the Constitution allows for same-sex couples to marry, effectively overturning remaining restrictions in place in states.

Prior to the ruling, 37 states and the District of Columbia had legalized gay marriage: Alabama, Alaska, Arizona, California, Colorado, Connecticut, Delaware, Florida, Hawaii, Idaho, Illinois, Indiana, Iowa, Kansas, Maine, Maryland, Massachusetts, Minnesota, Montana, Nevada, New Hampshire, New Jersey, New Mexico, New York, North Carolina, Oklahoma, Oregon, Pennsylvania, Rhode Island, South Carolina, Utah, Vermont, Virginia, Washington, West Virginia, Wisconsin and Wyoming.

LGBTQ HEALTH STATISTICS **

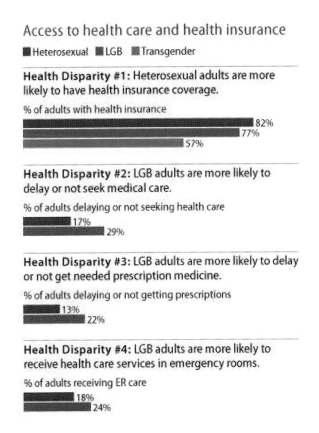

Access to health care and health insurance

■ Heterosexual ■ LGB ■ Transgender

Health Disparity #1: Heterosexual adults are more likely to have health insurance coverage.

% of adults with health insurance

82%
77%
57%

Health Disparity #2: LGB adults are more likely to delay or not seek medical care.

% of adults delaying or not seeking health care

17%
29%

Health Disparity #3: LGB adults are more likely to delay or not get needed prescription medicine.

% of adults delaying or not getting prescriptions

13%
22%

Health Disparity #4: LGB adults are more likely to receive health care services in emergency rooms.

% of adults receiving ER care

18%
24%

189

Impact of societal biases on physical health and well-being

■ Heterosexual ■ LGB ■ Transgender

Health Disparity #5: Heterosexual adults are more likely to report having excellent or very good overall health.

% of adults reporting excellent or very good health

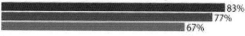

83%
77%
67%

Health Disparity #6: Lesbian and bisexual women are less likely to receive mammograms.

% of women receiving a mammogram in past 2 years

62%
57%

Health Disparity #7: LGB adults are more likely to have cancer.

% of adults ever diagnosed with cancer

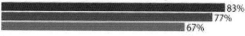

6%
9%

Health Disparity #8: LGB youth are more likely to be threatened or injured with a weapon in school.

% of youth threatened or injured with a weapon

5%
19%

Health Disparity #9: LGB youth are more likely to be in physical fights that require medical treatment.

% of youth in a physical fight requiring medical treatment

4%
13%

Health Disparity #10: LGB youth are more likely to be overweight.

% of youth who are overweight

6%
12%

Impact of societal biases on mental health and well-being

■Heterosexual ■LGB ■Transgender

Health Disparity #11: LGB adults are more likely to experience psychological distress.

% of adults experiencing psychological distress in past year

9%
20%

Health Disparity #12: LGB adults are more likely to need medication for emotional health issues.

% of adults needing medication for mental health

10%
22%

Health Disparity #13: Transgender adults are much more likely to have suicide ideation.

% of adults reporting suicide ideation

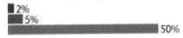
2%
5%
50%

Health Disparity #14: LGB youth are much more likely to attempt suicide.

% of youth reporting suicide attempts

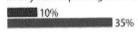
10%
35%

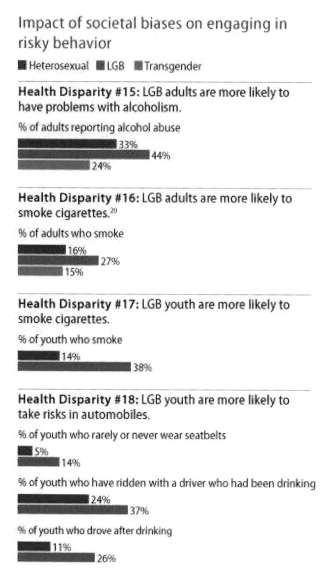

Impact of societal biases on engaging in risky behavior

■ Heterosexual ■ LGB ■ Transgender

Health Disparity #15: LGB adults are more likely to have problems with alcoholism.

% of adults reporting alcohol abuse

33%
44%
24%

Health Disparity #16: LGB adults are more likely to smoke cigarettes.[20]

% of adults who smoke

16%
27%
15%

Health Disparity #17: LGB youth are more likely to smoke cigarettes.

% of youth who smoke

14%
38%

Health Disparity #18: LGB youth are more likely to take risks in automobiles.

% of youth who rarely or never wear seatbelts

5%
14%

% of youth who have ridden with a driver who had been drinking

24%
37%

% of youth who drove after drinking

11%
26%

** Excerpts from Article by Jeff Krehely 2009 How to Close the LGBTQ Health Gap American Progress

As you can see by the statistics, members of the Gay community continue to experience worse health outcomes than their Straight counterparts. Due to factors like low rates of health insurance coverage, high rates of stress due to harassment and discrimination in the workplace and other areas of their lives, and a lack of easy access to the health care system, Gay people are at a higher risk for cancer, mental illnesses, and other diseases, and are more likely to smoke, drink alcohol, use drugs, and engage in other risky behaviors.

Other statistics have found that they are twice as likely to live and age alone, and many lack family support.

LGBT HEALTH DISPARITIES

According to the 1973 American Medical Journal, Homosexuality was listed as a Disorder in the *Diagnostic and Statistical Manual of Mental Disorders (DSM)*. It wasn't until December 3, 2012 that the American Psychiatric Association board of trustees approved the latest proposed revisions to the *Diagnostic and Statistical Manual of Mental Disorders*, what will now be known as the *DSM-5*.

This marks a historic milestone for people who are transgender and gender non-conforming, as their identities are no longer classified as a mental disorder.

It is now known as "Gender Dysphoria" to represent the emotional distress that can result from "a marked incongruence between one's experienced/expressed gender and assigned gender." This will allow for affirmative treatment and transition care without the stigma of disorder

Many physicians have abandoned the previous views and medical organizations around the country have tried to distance themselves from this relatively recent embarrassing history. Although gay rights have surges nationwide, the healthcare community is struggling to keep up.

As recently as the 1990's, nearly 1/5th of physicians in a California Survey endorsed homophobic views, and 18% reported not feeling comfortable treating gay or lesbian patients (Smith 2007).

194

Because of prior experiences of bias or the expectation of poor treatment, many Gay patients reported a reluctance to reveal their sexual orientation or gender identity to their health providers.

As shown by the statistical charts, Gay patients are more likely to have difficulty accessing health care and less likely to have health insurance.

In the 1990's the AIDS outbreak occurred and many Gay patients experienced an assumption by health providers that they were positive, regardless of any lab results.

Despite the change of Standard Precautions for infection control, there have been many in the gay community that experienced these painful assumptions, and discrimination from healthcare providers. The education has been unable to keep up with some healthcare staff personal religious beliefs, and prejudice, sadly.

No federal health survey includes a question on sexual orientation or gender identity, and only a few states ask respondents their sexual orientation or gender identity, severely limiting researchers' ability to fully understand the Gay patient's needs and hindering the development of public policies and programs that seek to improve the Gay population's health and well-being. Because of the lack of accurate data, it is virtually impossible to know how many people aging in America fit into this category.

Furthermore, many due to society pressure have referred to their partner as a "roommate", or "friend", and do not disclose their true sexual preference to health providers, otherwise known as "Coming Out".

The social stigmas and religious beliefs amongst healthcare professionals have created a sense of hostility and fear for many in the Gay community. The fear that all Gay people must have HIV/AIDS in the past created many unpleasant experiences for the patient seeking healthcare and treatments.

Most are seeking treatment for the most common of afflictions: high blood pressure, weight loss and hormone balance.

When a patient is positive with HIV/AIDS, it's been difficult to get rehabilitation centers and nursing homes to admit them, sometimes due to the prejudice of management. Recently, an HIV/AIDS patient had been admitted into a Skilled Nursing Center, and the staff refused to bath him, for fear of infection. Most irrationally, as all health personnel are to be using Standard Precautions (wearing gloves, etc.) on all patients, despite the diagnosis of the patient.

In the past, it was difficult for a Gay patient to know which healthcare providers were "gay friendly" or not.

Some states are attempting to change this by posting rainbow symbols on their signs and marketing collaterals, identifying those companies as "gay friendly."

196

Many of the newer and younger physicians are more open to the gay community, having grown up with those that identify themselves as gay.

Research shows that gay youths have a high rate of suicide attempts and homelessness. Complications of substance abuse can further contribute to depression, sexually transmitted diseases, and obesity.

The resistance of the healthcare community to provide education and compassion has caused some gay patients to refuse medical treatment and care, even when needed.

Older Gay individuals face unique challenges as they age. Most of them grew up in time periods of less social acceptance of the gay lifestyle and may harbor greater fear of stigma and discrimination than their younger counterparts.

TIPS FOR FINDING A GAY FRIENDLY HEALTH CARE PROVIDERS

When trying to find "Gay friendly" Health providers it's helpful to look for the rainbow sign on marketing collaterals, as well as word of mouth.

Call your insurance company and ask specifically for a primary care physician that is identified as Gay friendly. They may have a pride symbol as party of their profile, and the representative may not know what that means, so be persistent.

Talk with your peers or visit your local Gay community center. To find one near you, contact the website below:

http://www.lgbtcenters.org/ Center Link

The websites listed below can also be helpful:

www.glma.org   Gay & Lesbian Medical Association

www.aglp.org   Association of Gay & Lesbian Psychiatrists

www.healthfinder.gov/FindServices/Organizations/Organization.aspx?code=HR3450 Healthfinder.gov

www.pflag.org   Parent, Friends of Lesbians & Gays

www.outforhealth.org   Out for Health

http://www.hrc.org/resources/coming-out-to-your-doctor
Human Rights Campaign

Once you've found a potential good match, make sure to call the Office and ask if they have other gay patients. Also, ask about insurance plans they take, and any co-payments that you may be responsible for.

During the office visit, look for **Non-Discrimination Posters**, **Safe zone brochures, rainbow symbols**, or brochures for the **LGBTQ Patient**.

To determine if a health care provider is the best for you ask yourself the following questions:

- Did he/she seem at ease with you?
- Did he/she talk openly about your sexuality or gender identity?
- Could you have an open discussion?
- Were you able to be honest about partners, health issues, and habits?
- Did they suggest overall wellness suggestions?

When navigating the healthcare system as a Gay patient, make sure to get your **Advanced Directives** in place and in particular a **Health Care Surrogate Document** assignment. (See Chapter 4-5 for free access).

Having those documents in place and easily accessible will help the healthcare providers communicate with your loved ones in the event of a medical emergency. They will also ensure your wishes for care are honored. They are your best defense against any lingering prejudice and social discrimination that a healthcare staff member may have.

Although health education is trying to keep up with all the changes in equality in this county, it is difficult to remove years of prejudice from some health care providers and staff members.

The best Defense is a good Offense

 I would urge all to embrace the **Gay Friendly** health care providers that are available, get your annual physicals, and handle quickly any health concerns that arise.

Modern medicine is much more advanced than in years prior, and there are more medications and treatments available for any medical conditions that you or a loved one may experience.

Preparing for an "unplanned" medical event is essential in making sure that all of your loved ones get information about your condition, and that any and all of your wishes for care are honored.

I've witnessed many **Gay** patients that take their healthcare needs seriously, and with the right healthcare provider, a lot of worry and depression can be avoided.

Other Resources

www.nami.org/glbt (800) 950-6264 www.lgbthealth.net	**National Association of Mental Illness (NAMI)** **National Coalition for LGBT Health**
www.thetrevorproject.org (888) 340-8078	**GLBT Help Line**
(800) 850-8078	**LGBTQ Suicide Prevention Hotline**

CHAPTER 14

HOW LGBTQ COUPLES CAN PROTECT EACH OTHER AS THEY AGE

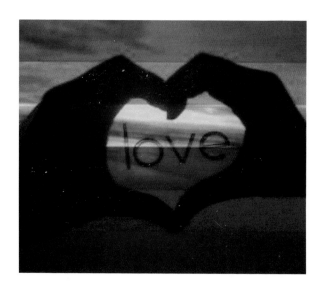

Marriage is about Love, Not Gender

STATES THAT ALLOW MARRIAGE EQUALITY**

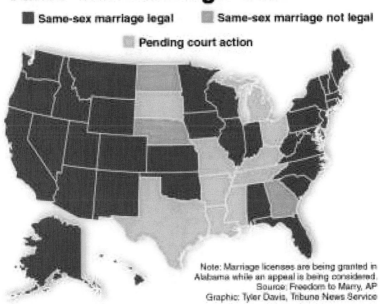

** Map from Academe Blog April 29, 2015

https://academeblog.org/2015/04/29/same-sex-marriage-urban-discontent-and-american-values/

LOVE STORIES

Older gay couples have lived in the shadows for many years and are now in many states able to marry and enjoy the privileges that strait couples enjoy.

Finally, they can come into the light and pronounce their love for each other!

Since many of them have lived as roommates, or friends, they are now finding new options for each other that were never previously available, such as health and life insurance coverage, disability and long term care insurance policies, and legal documents that have more protection than previously offered.

Once such couple I met we lovingly referred to as "the Annie's" as one was named Ann and the other Anna. They had lived together for over 35 years as roommates and partners and were now both in their 80's and beginning to need more care. They lived in a state that had not legalized marriage as of yet, however, were happy to take advantage of that when it became an option, and are now married.

The challenge arose when they needed more care, however, were legally recognized as single individuals, both with different types of care needs. One had a very low monthly income and qualified for the State Medicaid Home care assistance, however, had co-mingled money with her partner for many decades.

Her partner had a sizeable monthly income, and since their money had been in a shared bank account, automatically disqualifying her for that program.

The wealthier Annie had served our country, and only missed being eligible for the Aid & Attendance benefit by 1 day of service.

The biggest challenge in meeting their health needs within the scope of their financial situation was a case that has become more common than imagined. We did get an elder law attorney that was able to sort through their finances to eventually enable the one Annie to qualify for the Medicare Home Care program, after costly billable hours by his office.

My advice for roommates that are sharing accounts, is to establish a joint account for household bills, and keep any other finances separate for the sake of qualifying for any future care programs that usually require "legally single" individuals have their own accounts for verification.

It didn't matter that they referred to each other as "wives" when trying to qualify for state benefits. It was their current marital situation under the law that was recognized.

I'm happy to report they are now happily married and living in an assisted living facility that also accepted their cats.

These love stories are all over America, and are heartwarming to witness how they care for each other, in many cases for decades of time and adversity.

If you are in a "coupled" situation and are unmarried, keep your money separate, which is good advice for straight couples also.

Marriage is as much of a financial and legal binding arrangement, as a joining of two hearts and lives. Because of the financial and legal ramifications, it is always best to NOT co-mingle money, property and investments as a legally single person, regardless of your sexual preference.

I've known of gay couples that have bought homes or businesses together, and when the relationship broke up was a sticky legal mess, much like a divorce.

Always count the cost when entering into any financial situation with someone you love. Make sure you have the test of time, love and trustworthiness on your side.

WERE FINALLY MARRIED – NOW WHAT?

Congratulations, being a legally married couple now means in some cases, that the company will now allow the spouse to be covered on health, life and disability benefits. It also means that you get the same benefits and risks that the straight couples have experienced for years.

The best ways to protect each other financially and medically is to prepare for an "unplanned medical event". Healthcare costs in this country continue to rise each year, and individuals over 65 years of age now have a 70% chance of requiring some type of long term care. That can include home care help, assisted living, adult day care services or skilled nursing care.

The first thing to take care of is your Advanced Directives documents mentioned in Chapter 4, which are essential for healthcare providers to exchange information in case of an "unplanned medical event".

This means establishing each other as a Healthcare Surrogate or Proxy, depending on the state. A living will and power of attorney papers are also essential in the event decisions need to me made quickly.

Some Insurance providers have been planning for the time when gay couples would now be able to purchase long term care policies for each other. These are policies that will pay for care when needed, either at home or in a facility. Shop these policies to see if you can be able to purchase them.

There are couples that are depending financially on the money received for their home care from these policies, and are a great way to ensure that your savings are not depleted by an illness or need for additional care.
No one ever plans to get sick, have an accident, or land in a hospital, thus "unplanned event". However, patients that are prepared in this situation can weather the storm much better than others.

Having advanced directives, including health care surrogate paperwork can assist in an emergency in getting medical and financial updates, and any decisions that need to be made. It's the best way to protect each other from any prejudice any healthcare providers may have.

It's one thing to choose a Gay Friendly provider on an outpatient basis, but when thrown into a Hospital situation in an emergency, the better prepared you are, the better care you or your loved one will receive.

If you are living in a state where gay marriage has **NOT** been legalized, it's even more important to have your documents up to date in the event of an emergency. Anyone can get into a car accident, have a fall, or suddenly become ill. We are all human.

The **"HIPPA COMPLIANT"** defense goes right out the window if you have the Advanced Directive documents with you as a precaution. It's superman's kryptonite, if you will.

It's interesting to see the double standard applied even to our elderly gay population, who have already been through decades of discrimination with this country. It's heart breaking, but the sad reality of prejudice in its ugliest form.

Having this paper readily available in the event of an emergency can avoid the anguish of not being given information, or being "kept in the dark." This applies even to close friends also. In many areas of the country healthcare professionals haven't met or known any gay people, and those they may know that are, do not feel free to "come out", so it's helpful to not let them use their personal prejudice against you or a loved one in a medical emergency.

Physicians that have hospital privileges are an additional layer of protection in the event of a hospital emergency.

When a physician does not have hospital privileges, a hospitalist physician will assume care, and may or may not have access to a person's health history. Because of this, it's a good practice to attach to the Advance Directive paperwork, a copy of an insurance card, and a current medication listing, along with any allergies, for the healthcare professionals to use.

A primary care physician that is non- judgmental with hospital privileges can be an advocate, leader and protector in case there is a medical emergency. Also, they may include many preventative mental health therapies that can help any patients struggling with depression, shame, PTSD, substance abuse, or other medical conditions.

Now that you're a married couple, you get all the legal benefits, but still need to protect each other from the lingering prejudice that can exist in the healthcare industry.

The best defense is a good offense, therefore, having all necessary paperwork in place will hopefully ensure communication, better care, and a long and happy life with each other!

The websites listed below can be helpful:

www.glma.org Gay & Lesbian Medical Association

www.aglp.org Association of Gay & Lesbian Psychiatrists

www.healthfinder.gov/FindServices/Organizations/Organi
zation.aspx?code=HR3450 Healthfinder.gov

www.pflag.org Parents, Friends of Lesbians & Gays

www.outforhealth.org Out for Health

http://www.hrc.org/resources/coming-out-to-your-doctor
Human Rights Campaign

(See Chapter 1 for more physician websites)

To find a Financial Professional:

www.eapps.naic.org/forms/ipsd/Consumer_info.jsp
National Association Insurance Commissioners

To check the financial standing of a company:
www.adviserinfo.sec.gov
www.standardandpoors.com
www.ambest.com
www.moodys.com

Other Resources

www.nami.org/glbt National Association of Mental Illness (800) 950-6264

www.lgbthealth.net National Coalition for LGBT Health

GLBT Help Line (888) 340-8078
www.thetrevorproject.org

LGBT Suicide Prevention Hotline
(800) 850-8078

CHAPTER 15

FALL PREVENTION &

SAFETY TIPS

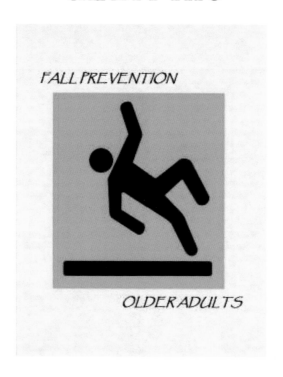

"Safety doesn't happen by Accident."

Author Unknown

THE FALL PREVENTION MOVEMENT

Despite falls being the leading cause of injuries in older adults, and injury related deaths, it wasn't until 2004 that this health issue began to get national attention.

The National Council on Aging launched the Falls Free® Initiative in 2005, which was a group of national and state agencies working together to address this issue and create solutions. Since then, it has gained a lot of awareness, and is increasingly swift with programs and education.

The end result s of all of these previous efforts has resulted in many fall prevention coalitions, and partnerships nationwide.

Although this has gained much advocacy and education, health providers are still struggling to change and improve the statistical outcomes of older adults that fall, and fall related injuries.

Consistently we are trying to adjust and change a population that is living longer, and resisting changes, even if they are for their own safety.

The best defense is knowledge, and the statistics highlight the importance of this movement to educate all older adults.

FALL RELATED INJURY STATISTICS*

In 2012, over 2.4 million older adults were treated in emergency departments for falls; more than 722,000 or 30% of these patients had to be hospitalized

(1). Every 29 min, an older adult in the United States dies from fall-related injuries

(2). Direct medical costs for fall injuries total over $30 billion per year in the nation and account for 6% of all medical expenditures for this age group

(3, 4). The risk of falling increases with age, and accelerates after age 85 years due to issues such as declining muscle strength, increased frailty, poor eyesight, and limited movement

(5). With an increased life expectancy among the growing baby boomer population, the problem of older adult falls has the potential to overwhelm resources required to address the needs.

Until 2004, the issue of older adult falls received little national attention in part due to its complexity and lack of readily available evidence-base interventions.

As a growing public health issue, it clearly needed a national effort to promote awareness and action. Since then, attention to the issue of older adult falls has gained significant momentum through the work of many stakeholders around the country, primarily led through the National Council on Aging's (NCOA) Falls Free® Initiative

(6). Launched in 2005, the Falls Free® Initiative brought together national and state agencies to collaboratively address older adult falls with evidence-based solutions; the authors of this article were leaders in the effort. The Falls Free® Initiative has been particularly successful in advocacy at the national level and in supporting the creation and development of state fall prevention coalitions and local collaborative efforts across the country. The purpose of this paper is to describe the steps taken to create the momentum around fall prevention and lessons learned that could be applied to supporting other older adult health-related issues. Steps include creating a national initiative; initiating advocacy efforts; and developing and supporting coalitions to increase awareness of the issue, promote evidence-based programs, institute evaluation, and implement policy and systems change.

* Statistical report from taken from
http://journal.frontiersin.org/article/10.3389/fpubh.2014.00194/full

FALLS IN OLDER ADULTS

The reason that this issue is so important is because falls in older adults is avoidable, and sometimes very easy to avoid. The sad reality is that many seniors that fall do not return to an independent life afterwards.

Falls Are Serious and Costly

- One out of five falls causes a serious injury such as broken bones or a head injury.
- Each year, 2.5 million older people are treated in emergency departments for fall injuries.
- Over 700,000 patients a year are hospitalized because of a fall injury, most often because of a head injury or hip fracture.
- Each year at least 250,000 older people are hospitalized for hip fractures.
- More than 95% of hip fractures are caused by falling, usually by falling sideways.
- Falls are the most common cause of traumatic brain injuries (TBI).
- Adjusted for inflation, the direct medical costs for fall injuries are $34 billion annually. Hospital costs account for two-thirds of the total.

WHAT CAN HAPPEN AFTER A FALL?

Many falls do not cause injuries. But one out of five falls does cause a serious injury such as a broken bone or a head injury. These injuries can make it hard for a person to get around, do everyday activities, or live on their own.

- Falls can cause broken bones, like wrist, arm, ankle, pelvic, and hip fractures.
- Falls can cause head injuries. These can be very serious, especially if the person is taking certain medicines (like blood thinners). An older person who falls and hits their head should see their doctor right away to make sure they don't have a brain injury.
- Many people, who've fallen, even if they're not injured, become afraid of falling. This fear may cause a person to cut down on their everyday activities. When a person is less active, they become weaker and this increases their chances of falling.[9]

WHAT CONDITIONS MAKE IT MORE LIKELY TO FALL?

Research has identified many conditions that contribute to falling. These are called risk factors. Many risk factors can be changed or modified to help prevent falls. They include:

- Lower body weakness
- Vitamin D deficiency (that is, not enough vitamin D in your system)
- Difficulties with walking and balance
- Use of medicines, such as tranquilizers, sedatives, or antidepressants. Even some over-the-counter medicines can affect balance and how steady you are on your feet.
- Vision problems
- Foot pain or poor footwear
- Home hazards or dangers such as
  - broken or uneven steps,
  - throw rugs or clutter that can be tripped over, and
  - No hand rails along stairs or in the bathroom.

Most falls are caused by a combination of risk factors. The more risk factors a person has, the greater their chances of falling.***

*** Statistics taken from www.cdc.gov/HomeandRecreationalSafety/Falls/adultfalls.html

Each year, one in every three adults ages 65 or older falls and 2 million are treated in emergency departments for fall-related injuries. And the risk of falling increases with each decade of life.

The long-term consequences of fall injuries, such as hip fractures and traumatic brain injuries (TBI), can impact the health and independence of older adults. Thankfully, falls are not an inevitable part of aging. In fact, many falls can be prevented. Everyone can take actions to protect the older adults they care about.

FALL PREVENTION TIPS

You can play a role in preventing falls. Encourage the older adults in your life to:

- <u>Get some exercise</u>. Lack of exercise can lead to weak legs and this increases the chances of falling. Exercise programs such as Tai Chi can increase strength and improve balance, making falls much less likely. Also, swimming can be an excellent option for safe movement.
- <u>Be mindful of medications.</u> Some medicines—or combinations of medicines—can have side effects such as dizziness or drowsiness. This can make falling more likely. Having a doctor or pharmacist review all medications can help reduce the chance of risky side effects and drug interactions.

- <u>Keep their vision sharp.</u> Poor vision can make it harder to get around safely. Older adults should have their eyes checked every year and wear glasses or contact lenses with the right prescription strength to ensure they are seeing clearly.
- <u>Eliminate hazards at home.</u> About half of all falls happen at home. A home safety check can help identify potential fall hazards that need to be removed

- or changed, such as tripping hazards, clutter, and poor lighting.

The following checklist can help older adults reduce their risk of falling at home:

- <u>Remove things you can trip over</u> (such as papers, books, clothes, and shoes) from stairs and places where you walk.
- <u>Install handrails and lights</u> on all staircases.
- <u>Remove small throw rugs</u> or use double-sided tape to keep the rugs from slipping.
- <u>Keep items you use often in cabinets</u> you can reach easily without using a step stool.
- <u>Put grab bars inside and next to the tub</u> or shower and next to your toilet.
- <u>Use non-slip mats in the bathtub</u> and on shower floors.
- <u>Improve the lighting in your home</u>. As you get older, you need brighter lights to see well. Hang lightweight curtains or shades to reduce glare. Motion detection lights are recommended.
- <u>Wear shoes both inside and outside the house.</u> Avoid going barefoot or wearing slippers. Wear sturdy, well fitting, low heeled shoes with non-slip soles.
- <u>Be aware of uneven surfaces</u> indoors and outdoors. Smooth out wrinkles and folds in carpeting. Step carefully.
- <u>Stairways should be well lit</u> from both the top and the bottom. Have easy to grip handrails installed along the full length of both sides of the stairs.

- <u>Take your time.</u> Get out of chairs slowly. Sit a moment before you get out of your bed. Stand and get your balance before you walk. Be aware of your surroundings.

BEST PRACTICES AFTER A FALL

Many older adults are embarrassed after they've had a fall, and are fearful of losing their independence at home. Falls are a natural part of the aging process and happen to almost all adults 85 years young and older.

The most important thing is to make sure nothing is broken or fractured, an x-ray or a call to the primary care physician is always recommended after a fall. Also, if there is any difficulty in walking after, physical and/or occupational therapy is usually helpful, even if it was only a minor fall. A doctor can order this Medicare Skilled Home Care up to four times a year for "Gait Strengthening", and is a good preventative way to maintain independence at home.

Most importantly, look at the prevention tips in a home, and don't be afraid to admit if a fall has occurred. The chances of one happening as we age are very likely, despite all of our best efforts.

FIRE PREVENTION & SAFETY TIPS

Most local city fire departments offer some community education on ways to prevent home fires and are a resource to ensure that one doesn't occur.

Lifetime Possibility after Age 65 that an Event will occur:

3% Major House Fire:

FACT~ There are 395,000 major house fires annually.

❖ Test smoke alarms monthly. Make sure everyone in the home can hear the smoke alarms. They save lives!

❖ If you smoke, smoke outside. Wet cigarette butts before throwing them out or bury them in sand. Never smoke in bed or if oxygen is used in the home.

❖ Give space heaters space. Keep them at least 3 feet (1meter) away from anything that can burn - including you. Shut off heaters when you leave or go to bed.

❖ Stay in the kitchen when frying food. Never leave cooking unattended. Wear form fitting short sleeves when cooking.

If a pan catches fire, slide a lid over it and turn off the burner. Don't cook is you are drowsy from alcohol or medication.

❖ Stop, drop, and roll. If your clothes catch on fire stop (don't run), drop gently to the ground, and cover your face with your hands. Roll over and over to put out the fire. If burned, use cool water for 3-5 minutes to cool the burn. Get medical help immediately.

❖ Plan and practice your escape from fire and smoke.

❖ Know your local emergency number. Ask if it is 9-1-1 or a different number. Have a telephone near your bed in case you are trapped by smoke or fire.

❖ Plan your escape around your abilities. Have necessary items near your bed, such as glasses, your walker, cane, or wheelchair.

SENIOR DRIVING STRATEGIES

When is it time to stop driving?

Are you dreading "the talk" with your parents or grandparents regarding their safety and the safety of others on the road?

You are not alone!

In October 2005, a 93 year old man struck a pedestrian in St. Petersburg, Florida, and did not notice the body hanging on his windshield until a tollbooth operator stopped him.

These kinds of situations highlight the risks of older drivers on the road and have led to calls for stricter state licensing policies for older drivers.

Studies have shown that physical and cognitive degeneration at older ages compromises a person's driving ability. Sometimes families aren't always aware that their elderly loved one has become a danger on the road.

Many elderly drivers are in denial of their personal deficiencies, and resist the decision to turn over the keys. The desire to remain independent for as long as possible is and innate human quality, that can be a huge obstacle to overcome.

These are the statistics about older drivers.

"In 2012 more than 5,560 older adults were killed and more than 214,000 injured in motor vehicle crashes. These statistics reveal that an average of 15 older adults killed and 556 injured in crashes every day." **

**Injury Prevention & Control: Motor Vehicle Safety
htty://www.cdc.gov/motorvehiclesafety/older_adult_drivers/

By the year 2025, drivers 65 and older will represent 25% of the driving population. The studies indicate that fatal crashes increase starting at age 75, and increase drastically after age 80 and beyond.

Lifetime Possibility after Age 65 that an Event will occur:

Severe Car Accident: 17%

FACT: Some 2.9 million motor vehicle accidents result in death or injury.

TIPS FOR DRIVING SAFELY

- ❖ <u>Exercise Regularly</u> to increase strength and motor skills.
- ❖ <u>Vision Maintenance.</u> Have your eyes checked regularly, and wear glasses and corrective lenses as required.
- ❖ <u>Drive only during daylight hours</u> and in good weather.
- ❖ <u>Plan your route</u> before you drive.
- ❖ <u>Leave a large distance</u> between other cars in front and behind yours.
- ❖ <u>Avoid Distractions</u> such as talking on a cell phones, music, texting, eating, and drinking.
- ❖ <u>Use Alternatives</u> to driving, such as family, friends, public transportation, and taxi cabs.

TAKING THE KEYS AWAY FROM A PARENT

"Parents can push our buttons because they sewed them on."

Author Unknown

Taking Car keys away from an older, unsafe driving can become equal to war. The fight to maintain independence is an instinctive human trait that is not to be trifled with.

So what can be done?

First and foremost, treat them with love, kindness, and respect, and as an adult.

These are some tips that have worked for some families:

❖ Appeal to their sensibility and longevity with their loved ones.
❖ Offer alternative solutions to their need to drive (free/low cost drivers), senior public transportation programs.
❖ Maintain their locational habits. Make sure that they can still get to their friends, church, shopping, and recreational activities.
❖ Recruit the primary care physician, religious authorities and/or senior services police department officers to enforce the need.

❖ **LAST RESORT** – Take the car to an alternative
   location. (Mechanic, Relative, Friend)

Ultimately, the safety of a loved one can't be underestimated
in this regard. There have been situations of elderly people
drowning after driving into boat ramps, into oncoming
traffic, and trees.

There are many cities that are offering Older Driver Safety
Evaluation Testing. Use these agencies when necessary to
determine the physical and cognitive capabilities of an older
driver.

Be prepared for a fight, but know that it is a worthwhile one!

CHAPTER 16

TAKING A BREAK FROM CAREGIVING; RESPITE RESOURCES

"It is so important as a caregiver not to become so enmeshed in the role that you lose yourself. It's neither good for you nor your loved one."

- Dana Reeve

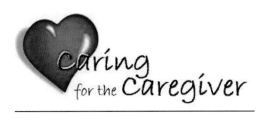

CAREGIVER RELIEF: WHY TAKE A BREAK

So many caregivers find themselves running on empty; selflessly taking care of a loved one's every need in a very "task oriented" way to the point that they may not even realize the fatigue and resentment they are feeling.

There are so many reasons to utilize respite care options, not simply to avoid burnout, but more importantly is that "Healthy Caregivers have Healthier Patients."

Where do I begin?

"START where you are, USE what you have, DO what you can."

Arthur Ashe, Professional Tennis Player

The simplest in home respite options are to use family members, friends, church groups, students from health colleges, and volunteers.

Many caregivers don't want to impose upon others however; many would prefer to help if they are asked. Furthermore, sometimes the patient may get tired of receiving care from the primary caregiver, and both can get a much needed "break" from each other.

Make a list of simple tasks that can be offered to people when they ask "do you need anything", and give them an answer: "Gee, I'd love to have help with laundry, run a doctor visit, pick up prescriptions, etc." Fill in an item off of your weekly task list.

There is a tool online that many families are using to distribute tasks to multiple caregivers called www.ecarediary.com. They have a message board, and the primary caregiver can put in tasks that they need help with, so that other family members can be notified and sign up. This can be an easier way than trying to remember that Mom/Dad has a need the primary caregiver may not be able to handle.

In home assistance can also come from Medicare Home Health providers such as physical therapists and nursing evaluations. Private duty home care agencies sometimes offer special packages that can be easily afforded.

In some states, Medicaid State Aid includes weekly private duty care staff to provide some health with the activities of daily living, Adult Day Care programs, and even Assisted Living financial assistance. To see if you qualify for Medicaid in your state, the process can begin online at www.medicaid.org (enter state).

In most cases, a case manager is assigned, and most interviews can be done over the phone, or in the home.

Out of the home respite options include Adult Day Centers, Residential Respite care, and Caregiver Support Groups. Assisted Living facilities often offer a 3-7 day Respite Stay program that can be free or reasonably priced, and key to attending family events, and maintaining a good life, work and balance in their role.

10 TIPS FOR TAKING BREAKS

1. Do something you enjoy. Get a latte. Take a bath. Phone a friend.

2. Communicate. Reach out to your support system and let them know how they can help. Let the one you're caring for know about the plans made.

3. Get outside. Actually going outdoors, and getting some fresh air, may work wonders.

4. Do some physical activity. I know some of you may be thinking you don't have time for that, but you will have more energy as caregiver if you do.

5. Take them regularly. And I'm talking like, every day. Even for a few minutes.

6. Call in for re-enforcement! Call a family member or a friend to ease your mind (and that guilt!) while you are 'off duty.'

7. Plan ahead. Some feel better actually scheduling breaks or certain activities into their schedule. That way everyone is aware and you can work around them.

8. Indulge. Get your hair or your nails done. Buy a new sweater. Go out for dessert. You deserve to treat yourself every once in a while.

9. Breaks before burnout. Get familiar with <u>the signs that burnout may be coming on</u>, and take a proper break and rest before it does.

10. Realize you are not superman/superwoman. No one can be all things to all people all of the time.

Research has found that breaks, taken regularly, actually contribute to the overall effectiveness of you as a family caregiver.

They allow you to refresh, refuel, and re-energize. They allow you to attend to life outside of being a family caregiver. And they also allow you to care, if only just a little, for yourself.

Part of being a family caregiver is also about caring for your own needs, to avoid sickness, chronic fatigue, exhaustion, burnout, resentment, anger and depression.

Self-care is not overrated. In fact, I would say it's the opposite. It's underrated. Looking after yourself, you will be able to look after others more successfully.

Some organizations that offer respite financial assistance are listed below:

www.aapd.com	American Association of People with Disabilities
www.archrespite.org	ARCH National Respite Network
www.caregiver.org	National Alliance for Caregiving
www.hospicefoundation.org	Hospice Foundation of America
www.nads.org	National Day Services Association
www.nmha.org	Mental Health America
www.nvcnetwork.org	National Volunteer Caregiving Network

Retired Military and their spouses often qualify for additional money to pay for care under the Aid and Attendance Benefit, which can pay up to an additional $2120.00 monthly to cover in home private duty caregivers, adult day care programs, and assisted living. If there are liquid assets over $80,000, (not including house or a car) then it's best to contact an Elder Law Attorney that specializes in Veteran Benefits to submit the application. However, if there are no liquid assets, or less than $80,000 (not including house or a car), then it's best to contact the local Veteran Service Officers (FREE) through the National Association of County Veteran Service Officers www.nacvso.org.

There are many other benefits that may be available through the VA Healthcare System including mental health counseling, social services and widows' benefits. To begin the application for the Veteran Healthcare System, go online at www.va.gov. You will need the veteran's DD214, social security number, and date of birth to get started.

Achieving balance as a Caregiver is essential in maintaining outside relationships, and good physical, emotional and mental health, as well as happier patients.

CHAPTER 17

RESOURCES FOR AGING HEALTHY, WEALTHY & WISELY

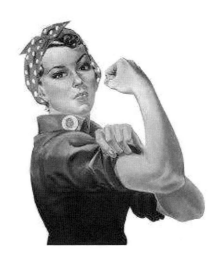

"Knowledge is Power."

Francis Bacon

IMPORTANT PHONE NUMBERS

AARP	800-424-3410
Abuse Hotline	800-96Abuse
Al-Anon – Alateen	800-344-2666
Alzheimer's Crisis	800-394-1771
America Council for the Blind	800-424-8666
American Kidney Foundation	800-424-8299
American Social Health	800-230-6039
Americans with Disabilities	800-350-4566
Arthritis Foundation	800-741-4008
Attorney Referral	800-342-8011
Cancer National	800-227-2345
Colon Cancer Alliance	888-422-2030
Domestic Violence	800-500-1119
Fraud Hotline	800-772-4258
Hospice National	800-658-8898
Insurance Consumer Hotline	800-342-2762
Internal Revenue Service	800-829-1040
Library for the Blind	800-226-6075
Medicaid Member Services	800-392-2161
Medicare Part B	800-392-2161
Medicare Information	800-638-6833
Office Controller	800-3362445
Ombudsmen	888-831-0404
Social Security Administration	800-772-1213
Senior Advisor Society	800-653-1785
The Senior Consumer	800-435-7352

<u>YOUR COMMUNITY RESOURCES</u>

Assisted Living Federation   703-894-1805
www.alfa.org

Eldercare Locator   800-677-1116
www.eldercare.gov

Leading Age   202-783-2242
www.leadingage.org

National Assoc. Home Care/Hospice   202-547-7424
www.nahc.org

National Assoc. Social Workers   202-408-8600
www.socialworkers.org

National Women's Health   800-994-9662
www.womenshealth.gov

NIH Senior Health   800-222-2225
www.nihseniorhealth.gov

SAGE   212-741-2247
www.sageusa.org

US Centers Disease Control   800-232-4636
www.cdc.gov/healthyliving/

YOUR FINANCIAL RESOURCES

National Assoc. Insurance   816-783-8500
www.naic.org

National Long Term Care Information   202-619-0724
www.longtermcare.gov

Pension Rights Center   202-296-3776
www.pensionrights.org

State Health Insurance Assistance   800-663-4227
www.shiptalk.org

US Dept. Veteran Affairs   800-827-1000
www.va.gov

US Social Security Administration   800-772-1213
www.ssa.gov

YOUR HEALTH RESOURCES

Alzheimer's Association   800-272-3900
www.alz.org

Centers for Medicare & Medicaid 800-633-4227
www.cms.gov

Family Caregiver Alliance   800-445-8106
www.caregiver.org

National Alliance for Caregiving 301-718-8444
www.cargiving.org

National Alliance for Hispanic Health 866-783-2645
www.hispanichealth.org

National Assoc. Geriatric Care Managers 520-881-8008
www.caremanager.org

National family Caregivers   800-896-3650
www.thefamilycaregiver.org

Aging with Dignity   888-594-7437
www.agingwithdignity.org

Caring Connections   800-658-8898
www.caringinfo.org

National Hospice   800-658-8898
www.nhpco.org

Long Term Care Ombudsmen   **202-332-2275**
www.ltcombudsman.org

HEALTH & WELLNESS WEBSITES

www.healthgrades.com	**Healthgrades**
www.ratemds.com	**Rate MD's**
www.vitals.com	**Vitals**
www.informedpatient.org	**Informed Patient**
www.hca.com	**HCA**
www.baycare.org	**BayCare**
www.va.gov	**Veteran Administration**
www.wellness.com	**Wellness**
www.healthcarefinder.gov	**Healthcare Finder**
www.medicare.org	**Medicare**
www.cms.org	**Centers for Medicare**
www.medicaid.org	**Medicaid**

SUMMARY

Aging in America can be a daunting challenge and learning how to navigate our healthcare system is tricky. The main message here is to research and plan ahead.

Having the "talk" with an aging loved one may be uncomfortable but will save grief, money and reactionary behaviors later.

Many seniors that are declining may stubbornly deny that they need help when they do, and it's up to caregivers to make sure not to allow the health and safety of their loved one to be in jeopardy.

Making sure they are safe and prepared can assist the healthcare professionals greatly in providing the best of care when our aging loved ones need it.

Understanding our healthcare system in our country can be an ever changing adventure, and the goal of this book is to provide as much information as possible.

Hopefully the information contained in this book will help us all to Age Healthier, Wealthier & Wisely!

AGING in AMERICA ORDER FORM

$19.99 per Copy

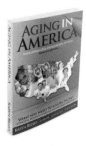

Check Payment to Elite Marketing
P.O. Box 7221
Seminole, FL 33775

Name: _____

Address: _____

City/State/Zip_____

Phone: _____Email_____

Large Quantity Orders at www.agingguidebook1.com

Email Author @ agingguidebook@gmail.com

www.agingguidebook1.com

This resource guide is meant to give an overall insight of the American Healthcare System, and a general overview of the key areas that may cause an impact on an aging person's healthcare experience.

If you'd like to receive information and resources that are personal to your specific situation, send an email to the following:

Email agingguidebook@gmail.com or

For more current and updated information, subscribe to www.agingguidebook1.com